Candida Albicans

Also by Leon Chaitow:

Fibromyalgia and Muscle Pain
High Blood Pressure
Natural Alternatives to Antibiotics

Candida Albicans

THE NON-DRUG APPROACH TO THE
TREATMENT OF CANDIDA INFECTION

Leon Chaitow

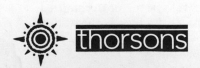

Thorsons
An Imprint of HarperCollins*Publishers*
77–85 Fulham Palace Road,
Hammersmith, London w6 8jb

The Thorsons website address is: www.thorsons.com

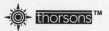

and *Thorsons* are trademarks of
HarperCollins*Publishers* Ltd

First published 1985
This revised edition published 2003

1 3 5 7 9 10 8 6 4 2

© Leon Chaitow 2003

Leon Chaitow asserts the moral right to
be identified as the author of this work

A catalogue record of this book is
available from the British Library

ISBN 0 00 715295 7

Printed and bound in Great Britain by
Creative Print and Design (Wales), Ebbw Vale

Contents

1 | Candida albicans and common health problems

Since the mid-1980s, it has become clear that an increasing number of common health problems, both physical and mental, might have a common cause – namely, the spread in the body of a yeast that lives in each and every one of us. Its name is *Candida albicans*, or Candida for short.

Since the first edition of this book (published in 1985), the major emphasis in my practice has involved people with Candida overgrowth as a part – often the major part – of their health problems, which commonly include symptoms of chronic fatigue, irritable bowel syndrome (IBS), allergies and fibromyalgia.

The scale of such problems worldwide has become increasingly apparent as a result of the stream of letters which continually arrives from readers of this book. Many contain phrases such as 'your book has changed my life', and often come with heartbreaking stories of desperate health situations which have been positively transformed (although not overnight) by the application of the methods and principles outlined in this book. While receiving such letters is truly humbling, the real credit should go to the pioneers of research into the subject of Candida, such as Dr C. Orian Truss of Alabama, USA, who first noticed what no one else seemed able to see, although it was staring them in the face. Because Candida yeast is present in everyone from the first few months of life, it tends to be overlooked by doctors seeking the causes of complex conditions which commonly involve multiple symptoms, including fatigue, allergies, IBS, 'brain fog' and muscle pain. Since this yeast is present in all of us to some extent, it seems that many doctors think that Candida could not possibly be causing the wide range of symptoms that are now linked to yeast overgrowth in so many people. This way of thinking has prevented sympathetic medical attention being given to Candida, except in rare conditions in which it proliferates to the extent of becoming life-threatening – something which happens in people whose defence mechanisms (immune system) has become weakened or deficient because of lifestyle, disease and/or drugs. Chronic Candida overgrowth can result in so many different symptoms that it has been renamed by many practitioners as Candida-related complex (CRC).[1]

A great many people suffer from a collection of symptoms due to the spread of Candida in their body. Usually, the conditions which are experienced are not severe enough to endanger life, but are certainly sufficient to produce a range of debilitating symptoms.

One of the most interesting summaries of the chronic ill health linked with Candida (particularly fibromyalgia and chronic fatigue syndrome) was presented at a conference on the subject in 1990 by Carol Jessop, MD, a leading physician from San Francisco.[2] She had studied the histories of over a thousand patients and discovered some alarming trends which can help us enormously to understand the way some health problems develop.

Among the most common symptoms reported by her patients were: chronic fatigue (100 per cent), cold extremities (100 per cent), impaired memory (100 per cent), frequent urination (95 per cent), depression (94 per cent), sleep disorder (94 per cent) and muscle aches (68 per cent). When patients were examined, among the most common findings reported by Dr Jessop was the presence of yeast infections (87 per cent). Of the 880 patients specifically tested for this,

82 per cent had yeast in their stool samples, and a further 30 per cent had parasites in these samples.

Among the most revealing of all were the findings when Dr Jessop investigated the symptoms experienced *before* their conditions became chronic: irritable bowel symptoms (89 per cent); recurrent childhood ear, nose and throat infections (89 per cent); 'constant gas' or bloating (80 per cent); endometriosis (65 per cent); constipation (58 per cent); heartburn (40 per cent); recurrent sinusitis (40 per cent); and recurrent bronchitis (30 per cent).

Most of the infections (ear, nose, throat, sinus, bronchitis, endometriosis) were almost certainly treated with course after course of antibiotics – the significance of which to the 'yeast connection' and digestive distress will become clear in later chapters.

Do you have a Candida problem?

Over the past few years, the following cluster of signs, symptoms and medical history indicators has been described by many practitioners as being present in people with chronic Candida problems.

1 The presence for at least two months of at least two digestive symptoms bad enough to cause you to change your diet or take medication such as:
    • constipation and/or diarrhoea
    • bloating
    • indigestion
    • heartburn/reflux
    • food sensitivities or allergies.

2 Constant or periodic feelings of profound ('unnatural')

fatigue, and difficulty in concentrating ('brain fog')
that is severe enough to affect the way you function.

3 One or more of the following: a sense of hopelessness,
anxiety, unnatural irritability, acne, migraine,
widespread muscular pain, cystitis, vaginitis, thrush,
menstrual problems, premenstrual tension.

4 A history of antibiotic use in excess of two courses
in any one year before the development of symptoms
(or the use of steroid medication or immune-
suppressing drugs for a lengthy period of time
(weeks rather than days).

For Candida overgrowth to be considered as the main
causative feature of these symptoms, other medical conditions need to be ruled out as causes (although Candida
overgrowth may coexist with any of these), such as:

• inflammatory bowel disease (colitis, for example)
• parasitic infection, such as *Giardia*
• bacterial overgrowth in the intestines
• hypothyroidism
• hypoadrenalism (Addison's disease).

Why does yeast spread?

To understand the way in which such a wide range of symptoms could result from the effects of a yeast that lives in
all of us, we need to first appreciate those factors which
encourage yeast to spread.

In most people, there is an uneasy 'truce' or balance
between the body and the yeasts that live inside it. Over
many thousands of years, a balance has been struck, allowing

yeast to live and thrive while presenting no problems to its host, the body, as long as the yeast confines itself to specific areas. Should it grow beyond these sites, the defence capability of the body – represented by the immune system in general and white blood cells in particular – will attack and destroy these overgrowing yeast. The mucous lining of the digestive tract, when it is healthy, provides a physical barrier to prevent the spread of yeast and waste products through it. This mucous membrane also contains and secretes protective substances that can destroy invading yeast.

An added defence comes from the 'friendly bacteria' living inside us (mainly in the digestive tract). We give these friendly bugs somewhere to live (as well as food) in return for which they provide us with various services, one of which is control of undesirable visitors, such as yeast. (These defences are covered later in this book, in our search for an understanding of candidiasis.)

At this stage, we should simply recognize that *when it is healthy*, the body possesses a number of efficient defence capabilities to deal with toxins, undesirable bacteria and yeasts, should any of them intrude into areas where they might cause problems.

But when, due to any of a number of possible causes (discussed later), our defences against Candida is deficient or weakened, the yeast has a chance to spread to areas normally out of bounds. If, at the same time, the foods that the yeast thrives on (such as sugar) happen to be in plentiful supply, an explosion of Candida activity can occur.

This situation – weakened defences and nourishment for Candida – is precisely the combination of factors that has been identified as having become widespread in Western society over the past 25 to 30 years.

The introduction of broad-spectrum antibiotics, the contraceptive pill and the widespread use of steroid medication (such as cortisone) have all played their part in Candida's spread. In addition, the increased use of sugar and sugar-rich foods has provided the yeast with just the sustenance it loves. This is the unfortunate combination of factors lying at the root of the problem for many people.

A careful look at the nature of the enemy is necessary, together with consideration of those factors and circum-stances which allow it to multiply, and what the consequences of such a proliferation might be. This will allow us to consider methods of controlling Candida, the brighter side of our sorry situation, for it seems unlikely that the causative elements of the 'yeast explosion' are going to go away. The fact that control is possible in the majority of cases is the good news.

Yeast is not always the cause

It is important to understand that the conditions listed above (such as irritable bowel, bloating, fatigue) are not always the result of Candida infection. However, it is true that all of these can be partly or entirely a result of candidiasis. It is the view of those practitioners now aware of the possibility of Candida's involvement in common disease problems of this sort that, when a combination of such symptoms appears in a person with no other obvious causes apparent, then Candida should be considered a prime suspect.

Unlike many infections and infestations, it is not easy (but not impossible) to test accurately for the presence of Candida. This is because, as already stated, Candida is present to some extent in all of us, which makes looking for it as pointless as searching for mice in a granary – it is always there. But to what extent, and how much is it involved in producing the symptoms?

Testing for Candida

Candida albicans (and other yeasts) are so common in stool cultures that their presence is often ignored by microbiologists. Medical researchers have highlighted the difficulty of assessing purely from tests whether Candida is active, even when it is known to be in an advanced stage of overgrowth.[3]

So what tests appear to be the most helpful – as none are perfect – in assessing the presence or absence of yeast overgrowth?

1 Culturing stool samples can be helpful in identifying specific strains of yeast as well as their quantities, but this is not a foolproof method since assessment depends on the particular sample submitted for analysis and, sometimes, people with known Candida overgrowth can produce stools containing relatively low levels of yeast. Faecal culturing has been shown to give 25 per cent false-negative results – that is, people with known yeast overgrowth can wrongly (in one in four negative tests) be assumed to be clear of the organism. And, since everyone has *some* yeast in the intestines, a positive test does not necessarily tell you that it is the cause of the symptoms being experienced. Nevertheless, these tests can be useful because, when they find high levels of Candida (or other yeasts), they can identify particular strains and also test these to see what medications (drugs and herbs) they are sensitive to. An additional advantage of the stool analysis is that it can identify the presence of parasites and pathogenic bacteria which might be causing or aggravating symptoms.

2 Gut fermentation tests involve a blood sample being taken before and after a sugar dose is taken on an empty stomach. The test assesses the amount of

alcohol (ethanol, methanol) produced by yeast in an hour. The amount found in the blood gives an indication of the level of yeast activity.

3 Gut permeability tests show whether there has been a change in the way the lining of the intestines protects the bloodstream from absorbing undesirable substances. This is not a measure of Candida itself because there are many other causes of increased permeability ('leaky gut'). However, one of the main causes of this is yeast overgrowth.

4 The bloodstream can be assessed for the presence of Candida antibodies. This test has been shown to give some false-negative results (no antibodies noted even though Candida is present). Another problem with this test is that it does not tell you what is happening now because antibodies may be present due to yeast overgrowth activity some time previously.

5 Tests can be done to see whether you are a secretor or non-secretor. We all have a blood type – A, B, AB or O – and most people (about 75–80 per cent) secrete minute amounts of chemical markers of their blood type into their normal secretions (such as saliva or mucus). The 20–25 per cent or so of those who are non-secretors, irrespective of their blood type, are known to have a greater tendency to infections of all sorts, and of yeast in particular. Women with recurrent vulvovaginal candidiasis, for example, are much more likely to be non-secretors. In addition, non-secretors handle sugars less efficiently than secretors, adding to the likelihood of yeast overgrowth.[4] A further aspect of this tendency shows that people who have type O blood, particularly if they are non-secretors, are far more likely to develop oral candidiasis.[5]

6 A person's health history (such as antibiotic use) and the way their symptoms respond to simple treatment strategies (cutting sugar intake, for example) can be an accurate way of confirming Candida activity as a factor in symptom production. A self-assessment questionnaire (*see Chapter 4*) provides a dependable guide as to whether or not Candida is currently active. This suggests that the way to prove that a condition (or cluster of conditions occurring together) is the result of Candida is to use a treatment that would reduce yeast activity. If the symptoms then improve markedly, or disappear altogether, such 'proof' that yeast was at least part of the cause would be difficult to contest.

Candidiasis is one of the few instances where the treatment of a health problem is, in fact, the main means of diagnosis. The initial suspicion that results in the treatment being started relies upon recognizing the sort of symptoms that suggest the presence of Candida as well as an awareness of those factors that influence its development and behaviour.

A careful background history which looks at previous and current medical treatment and drug usage, as well as diet and stress factors, will give clear signs of the likelihood, or otherwise, of Candida being a possible culprit.

It is these areas that we will explore to formulate a series of recommendations for the control of Candida and for the prevention of its accompanying complications.

Candidiasis is rapidly becoming so widespread as to constitute an epidemic, especially (as we will see), but not entirely, among women. The potentially disastrous health damage caused by the interaction between our bodies and a yeast that is usually easily tolerated and controlled is one of the complications of civilization. The failure, thus far, by all but a handful of doctors to recognize the situation is tragic, as the degree of human suffering involved is enormous. Prevention is not difficult, and control, while a slow process (taking months, not years), is not beyond the limits of any intelligent person.

The major credit for the unravelling of this mystery belongs to one man, who recognized that what he was seeing in his own patients had worldwide importance. Dr C. Orian Truss, of Birmingham, Alabama, will be remembered for his work in this field by hundreds of thousands of grateful people. His masterly investigation and research, conducted in a normal medical practice, show how important simple observation is in the quest for knowledge and the understanding of humanity's ills. Truss first set about diligently assembling his evidence, which he presented in a scientific journal. He then went back to his task of investigation. Over a period of years, his excellent clinical results in treating an enormous range of diseases – from acne to schizophrenia and what appeared to be multiple sclerosis – were so impressive that the world began to beat a path to his door. Dr Truss has written his own history of this research and of the whole story of Candida in his book *The Missing Diagnosis*.[6]

That book, and the excellent book on the same subject by another renowned American practitioner, Dr William Crook, entitled *The Yeast Connection*, both suggest for their attack on yeast the use of an antifungal drug called nystatin. They also suggest other methods, including nutrition and desensitization. This present book, however, will not attempt to echo such a drug approach, but will present non-drug alternatives to the use of nystatin. This is not to say that nystatin and other antifungal drugs should never be used, only that, in most cases, there are other, apparently safer ways of restoring the competence of the body to fight the yeast itself. There are sound reasons for trying to find anti-Candida alternatives (as will be explained in later chapters), including many naturally occurring nutrients which enhance the control of the wildly proliferating yeast without producing resistant strains, a problem now thought likely when nystatin is used for long periods. This is the only reason this book has needed to be written for, in every other way the two books mentioned on the previous page are excellent and valuable contributions to the literature of health.

We need now to take a closer look at the nature of the enemy, what makes it active and how to recognize such activity. Only then will we begin to learn how to deal with it.

REFERENCES

1 Stretch E. 'Clinical manifestations of HIV infection in women', *J Naturopath Med* 1992; 3(1): 12–19
2 *Fibromyalgia Network Newsletters* October 1990–January 1992
3 *The Lancet* 1987; January
4 Chaim W. 'Association of recurrent vaginal candidiasis and secretory ABO and Lewis phenotype', *J Infect Dis* 1997; 176(3): 828–30
5 Burford-Mason A. 'Oral carriage of *Candida albicans*, ABO blood group and secretor status in healthy subjects', *J Med Vet Mycol* 1988; 26(1): 49–56
6 Truss C. *J Orthomolec Psychiatry* 1980; 9(4): 287–301

2 | Candida and your defence systems

Candida infection (overgrowth) is increasing dramatically. Reports show that systemic (in the bloodstream) infections with Candida in the USA increased by up to nearly 500 per cent between 1980–89, with Candida accounting for 10 per cent of all organisms isolated from blood in hospitals.[1] The figures since then are bound to be even higher, and it is extremely important that we understand how to help the body protect itself from yeast overgrowth.

When we are ill, we have symptoms, and few symptoms are pleasant. But the symptoms are often signs that the body is fighting the actual cause of the condition. For example, if you have an infection, your temperature usually goes up, a clear sign that your immune system is fighting the infection. It is important to learn to understand symptoms and not to fight them, but to deal with the reason they are there. Another example would be the multiple symptoms of digestive distress, ranging from heartburn to bloating, constipation and/or diarrhoea. There are medications which will relieve these symptoms, although often only for a short time, but such medications will not deal with the underlying causes and often make matters worse in the long run.

There is one constant trend, even when we are unwell – that is, the body's self-healing tendency. Your many interacting body systems (including the immune system) and functions are constantly striving for balance, for normality – a process known as homoeostasis. Cuts heal, breaks mend, infections are overcome (usually without any outside

help); diarrhoea and vomiting, unpleasant as they undoubtedly are, are how the body gets rid of undesirable material
from inside itself.

So the message that needs to be heard is that symptoms
need to be understood so that we can learn what *causes*
them, not what can mask them. And we need to deal with
the many things we do which can aggravate and strain the
defence systems of the body to allow a chance for healing
and recovery.

Where infection is concerned, the ideal outcome is that
the bacteria, virus or yeast is contained and overwhelmed by
the homoeostatic defences of the body. Unfortunately, when
your homoeostatic mechanisms have to deal with too many
demands at the same time, they may not always be able to
achieve that outcome. Take, for example, someone who:

1 is not getting enough essential vitamins and/or
   minerals in the diet, and/or

2 is eating a poor diet loaded with refined carbohydrates
   and sugars, and/or

3 is not getting adequate exercise, and/or

4 has picked up a viral or yeast infection which never
   seems to quite go away, and/or

5 is not sleeping well, or getting enough exercise, and/or

6 is under work and/or emotional stress, and/or

7 has a slight hormonal imbalance, and/or

8 has a history of antibiotic use, and/or

9 is taking the contraceptive pill.

Each of these 'problems' (stresses), and others, may be relatively minor and could probably be eliminated by eating more sensibly, exercising more, ensuring a better exercise and sleep pattern, doing something positive about the emotional stress, or getting advice and treatment for the hormonal, viral and yeast problems. But, if nothing is done and these various adaptive demands (and others) continue, the body's defence and repair systems eventually become so overloaded that chronic symptoms start to appear.

And, of course, whatever emotional stress, nutritional deficiencies and acquired toxicities, and biomechanical stresses there may be (poor posture, tense muscles, poor breathing habits) that are added to this 'load', all are coped with in the context of the unique genetic characteristics with which each of us is born (*see notes on blood types and secretor status in Chapter 1, page 8*).

It seems that some people have inborn abilities to handle some of the 'stress' load more efficiently than others so that the symptoms, and their severity, that emerge from similar stress burdens will not be the same from one person to another.

What's the solution?

One of two things needs to be done:

1 There is a need to stop and reverse the factors which are causing the adaptive demands that are overloading the body's ability to cope;

2 There is also a need to provide help to the repair and support systems of the body to allow them to more efficiently handle the load they are coping with.

These changes need to take account of the person's unique characteristics and personal history (including their medical history). If the right changes are made, the homoeostatic defence systems should be able to begin to work more efficiently again to detoxify, fight infection, rebuild and repair, and symptoms should gradually ease. Some of the actions needed to help in recovery from a Candida overgrowth might involve:

1 ensuring optimal nutrition (removing tasty toxins and increasing nutritionally whole foods), and/or

2 a need to learn to handle stress differently, and/or

3 taking specific action to deactivate yeasts or other organisms, and/or

4 rebalancing hormonal status and the chemistry of the body (such as vitamins, minerals, trace elements, amino acids), and/or

5 detoxification of the system, particularly the liver, and/or

6 helping to heal the lining of the intestines, which may have been damaged by overgrowth of yeast, and/or

7 whatever else that may be needed to help reduce the adaptive demands that are overloading the homoeostatic systems.

About Candida

Candida albicans is a member of the yeast family. Strictly speaking, it is a member of a subgroup of the family of organisms known as fungi (or moulds). Yeasts live virtually everywhere on the planet and can derive their nutrients from most organic sources. This means anything that is alive, or has been alive, can support yeasts – whether animal or plant. Rather than having roots like other plants, yeasts can derive their nutrients via the enzymes they produce. Given the right conditions for growth and replication, yeast is capable of almost explosive growth, as anyone who has made bread will know.

Roger Williams, Nobel prize-winning scientist, stated that if a single yeast cell is given a highly favourable environment, with a good assortment of nutrients and the correct temperature, it can, within 24 hours, produce a colony of over 100 yeast cells.[2] At that rate of reproduction, Williams calculated, within one week, one cell could turn into a yeast colony weighing one billion tons.

The fact that this has not happened, and is not likely to happen, is solely because the environment is seldom ideal for any creature on earth, least of all for yeast. It does, however, highlight a very pertinent point in our understanding of the Candida problem: Candida is a yeast which lives inside of you and me and, as far as is known, every other adult on earth and most children as well. It seldom takes over our entire body but, when it does, the consequences are horrific. It can only achieve such a state if the environment for it is excellent and if the defence mechanisms that the body has to control its spread are weakened or absent. This can happen, for example, in advanced immune-deficiency situations, such as in AIDS.

As Williams pointed out, in Nature, yeast cells are almost always hampered by imperfect or inadequate environmental conditions. Were it not so, they would have engulfed the earth long ago. The same fact controls the colonies of Candida (and other yeasts) that live in and on you and me.

UNINVITED RESIDENTS OF THE BODY

Candida is usually a resident of the digestive system, largely in the lower end of the intestines. It also tends to occupy sites in the vaginal regions and on the skin, without causing any symptoms when general health and immune function are good.

Research has shown that most people have antibodies to Candida. The presence of these antibodies indicates that the individual's immune system has, at some time, been challenged to respond to the presence of the yeast. Dr Truss states that, by the age of six months at the latest, Candida is living in, or on, at least 90 per cent of people, as evidenced by a positive skin-test reaction when extracts of Candida are injected just under the skin.[3] This reaction shows that there has been a previous presence of the yeast to which the body has developed defensive antibodies.

The fact that yeast lives in all of us, and yet many people sail through life with no apparent ill effects, indicates that we have learned to cope with our uninvited yeast passengers. Unlike certain other minute creatures that live in our digestive tract and which serve a useful purpose, such as *Lactobacillus acidophilus* (which helps in the breakdown of food and in the synthesis of some of the B vitamins), there is no symbiotic (mutually beneficial) relationship with Candida. There is no trade-off whereby a 'room' is given in exchange for some useful function. So Candida is a pure and simple parasite – a freeloader. This is perhaps inevitable, given the multitude of opportunistic microscopic creatures in both the animal and vegetable kingdom. Most, if not all, plants and animals enjoy similar relationships with bacteria and fungi. Some of these relationships are symbiotic and good for both parties, while others are distinctly one-sided.

So Candida, for all the musical sound of its name, is an unwelcome squatter in your body and represents a potential danger. Once we know what sort of situation removes or reduces the ability of your body's defence systems to control it naturally, and what gives Candida the chance to proliferate, we will begin to understand what needs to be done to contain it when it gets out of hand and starts producing health problems.

It may be that we cannot actually stop yeast from taking up residence in the body, but we can certainly find ways to confine its activities to a small and relatively safe part of the premises.

The way the body defends itself

We need to understand some aspects of the body's amazing defensive capability. It has long been observed that people who survive certain infections seldom suffer from the same disease again. This is because they develop antibodies to the infecting organism. Apart from achieving specific resistance to various disease-causing microorganisms, the immune system plays a vital role in other biological reactions. In relation to infection, we have essentially two systems of defence. One is based on the thymus gland (which lies just below the breast bone), which produces what are called T cells. Another is part of the immune system and is made up of one type of white blood cells called B cells. These protect you from most bacterial invaders and some viral infections. By producing molecules called antibodies, the B cells neutralize many potential enemies. The two systems, together making up the surveillance and protection agency of the body, work in harmony although the thymus, it is thought, takes the leading role.[4]

THE BODY'S FRONT-LINE DEFENDERS

The white blood cells, which act as the soldiers in the front line of the battle, are manufactured mainly in the marrow of the long bones of the body. Some of these are turned into T cells by the influence of hormones from the thymus gland. • Other white blood cells become what are called lymphocytes. Anything that trics to get into the bloodstream or the interior of the body has to face the T and B cells, and their powerful ability to neutralize foreign substances or organisms. If a B cell senses a foreign organism, it produces antibodies that are specific to that invader. At the same time, other B cells are alerted to the alien presence, which causes them to manufacture antibodies to destroy the enemy.

It is believed that there are in excess of a million different kinds of antibodies in the bloodstream. As they are manufactured and deployed against the intruder, the lymphocytes go into action with other white blood cells to dispose of the debris and waste products of the battle between the intruder and the body. Thus, a condition such as influenza is self-limiting, with the fever and the symptoms of aching representing the intense activity going on in the body to deal with the invading virus, as well as the effects of the resulting toxicity of the breakdown products of the battle.

When T cells discover an invading organism, whether this is a virus or a fungus such as Candida (or even a mutant cancer cell), they produce substances called lymphokines, which can kill microorganisms (or cancer cells). One such lymphokine which has received much attention is interferon. Lymphokines can also call up assistance from powerful allies in this battle called macrophages, which can eliminate microorganisms and tumour cells by literally swallowing them whole. Sometimes, the T cells act as 'helper' cells to the B cells in their production of antibodies to fight off the invaders. They can also act as 'suppressor' cells to stop a defensive process from getting out of hand, when there may be a danger that the B or T cells may attack friendly tissues in the body (which is more likely to happen if the person is a non-secretor; see Chapter 1, page 8 for a brief description of this phenomenon).

What if the immune system is inefficient?

When for any one of a number of reasons (which we will consider in a later chapter) the immune system becomes weakened, we say that the person is immunodeficient, or has a poor immune response. It is when these valiant fighters – the T and B cells – and the macrophages and their various assistants are in a weakened state that silent 'squatters' in the body can become free of the constraints that the defence system normally imposes and spread to areas beyond their normal limits. When this happens, a vast array of problems and symptoms can arise.

The immune defence system, with its checks and balances, may become disrupted to such an extent that the condition now known simply by the initials AIDS may occur. The initials stand for acquired immunodeficiency syndrome and, in this condition, it is the T cells (from the thymus gland) that function inadequately. Indeed, the ratio between the helper and suppressor cells becomes so altered that there is an excess of suppressor cells, in contrast to the situation in normal health. Much of the research into the treatment of immune-related conditions focuses on methods to enhance the function of the thymus gland so that it can produce a balanced and adequate supply of active T cells. Among the nutrient factors which can also achieve this are vitamin C and the amino acid arginine.

How do you 'catch' Candida?

The short answer is that you seldom catch or acquire yeast infections from an external source, although new strains can be introduced via sexual contact, since you have Candida all the time!

A leading medical researcher into Candida activity describes what usually happens as follows:

The most important source of Candida species in human disease is endogenous [it comes from inside you]: candidiasis arises in people who are predisposed because of illness, debility or local reduction in resistance to overgrowth *of their own yeast flora.*[5]

The evidence of much research is that about half the *healthy* population (no illness or symptoms) has Candida yeast in their mouths, easily assessed by means of a swab sample.[6] Levels of Candida in the intestines of *healthy* individuals are described by researchers as 'high' – over 50 per cent – and, in ill people, especially where immune function is weakened, it is closer to 80 per cent.[7] Candida in the vagina is found in approximately 20 per cent of healthy women and, when there is also vaginitis (inflamed tissues) present, the levels are much higher – around 60 per cent (but not 100 per cent as many cases of vaginitis are caused by other organisms, such as *Trichomonas*).[5]

So, we can see that when the immune system is in a weakened state, not only do yeast infections become more frequent, but the infecting agent may not need to be acquired from the outside, as it may quietly be biding its time in small amounts in your mouth or digestive tract, waiting for your defences to drop (due to stress, infection, dietary indiscretions or any of a host of other factors). If this happens, the ever-present, opportunistic yeast will seize the opportunity to slip through the defence barriers and advance to areas previously closed to it.

This simplistic picture of what can happen contains the essential facts. Your body is self-healing. If this self-healing ability (known as homoeostasis) is weakened or overwhelmed, organisms such as yeasts which are already inside you can spread and cause havoc.

The solution to this scenario is twofold:

1 reduce the yeast (or other invading organism) activity, and
2 improve defence and self-healing potentials.

Some consequences of yeast overgrowth

We know that before it becomes invasive, the yeast (Candida) changes from a simple yeast to an aggressive mycelial fungus. In this altered form, Candida has characteristics that make it more dangerous, including a root structure which allows it to penetrate through the mucosal barriers of, say, the digestive tract. This can lead to a variety of harmful consequences because of easier access of toxins and breakdown products of digestion directly into the bloodstream (*see Chapter 4 for more detail*).

Research by Dr Truss[8] indicates that many of the toxic effects seen with Candida activity are the result of its ability to manufacture, under appropriate conditions, the substance acetaldehyde. Truss found that this well-known toxin can produce both the clinical and laboratory characteristics of Candida infection. Having analysed the amino acid profiles of affected individuals to arrive at this finding, Truss maintains that the symptoms of chronic yeast infection can be explained in terms of a toxin, which common strains of Candida have been shown to produce in the laboratory. This provides the chemical link between normal yeast fermentation and the metabolic abnormalities found in susceptible patients. Dr Truss stresses that it is highly probable that the symptoms experienced by many Candida sufferers relate directly to the ability of yeast to ferment sugar into acetaldehyde in the body.

As explained in Chapter 1, there are now tests which take advantage of this ability and which can measure any rise in blood alcohol levels after a 'sugar loading' in which alcohol (such as acetaldehyde) is measured after swallowing a specific amount of sugar on an empty stomach. However, this 'gut fermentation' test is not foolproof for a number of reasons, including the fact that other organisms, including certain bacteria which can live in the gut, can ferment sugar. But taken together with the person's history and symptoms, it can provide a strong indication of yeast activity.

Some laboratory technicians performing these tests (and many practitioners involved in treating chronic candidiasis) report being able to smell the alcohol resulting from eating sugar in people who never drink alcohol at all. In my own experience, I have treated individuals for candidiasis who have shown high levels of alcohol in their bloodstream despite not having consumed any alcohol.

Amalgam fillings and immune suppression

There is some evidence that immune system depression can result from mercury toxicity in the body as a result of amalgam fillings in teeth.[9] A number of researchers have shown that there are several ways in which this highly toxic metal is able to penetrate the body, with a specific, harmful effect on the immune system. There is also evidence that this can be linked to the spread of Candida activity. An increasing number of dentists are now helping affected individuals by removing mercury amalgam fillings and replacing them with either a composite or gold filling. However, it must be stressed that research into the relationship between mercury from dental fillings and health problems in general, and Candida involvement in particular, is incomplete. Yet, there is almost certainly a connection, and it is worth considering alternative choices for fillings other than amalgams that contain mercury.

The replacement of existing fillings may be required in cases where a connection can be demonstrated between a person's health and measurable mercury toxicity. The use of supplemental amino acid compounds, such as glutathione, and of vitamin C can help to ease mercury deposits from the body. If you have a Candida problem (with or without other bacterial overgrowth or gut parasites), a clue as to whether or not mercury may be affecting you can be gathered from your answers to the following questions – as well as testing for the presence of heavy metals such as mercury in your system – involving, among other things, measuring the levels of mercury vapour in the mouth as well as analysing sweat, urine and hair (and sometimes blood) by a suitably trained physician, nutritionist, naturopath or homoeopath:

- Do you have mercury (amalgam) fillings in your teeth?
- Is your skin sensitive to contact with metals such as nickel?
- Do your symptoms include some which are regarded as involving your nervous system, perhaps associated with visual symptoms or muscular weakness or tremor?
- Do you suffer from 'brain fog' – poor concentration and short-term memory?
- Do you have a tendency toward allergies and food intolerances/sensitivities?

If you answer 'yes' to the first and to any of the other questions, then mercury in particular and/or other toxic metals (for example, cadmium and lead) may well be part of your problem, and you should consider investigating this further.[10]

Other factors which encourage Candida spread

Although in Chapter 3 we will look at how Candida gets out of hand, it is worth adding here some information on the most common reasons for the spread of this yeast. Hints have already been given so far about the role of sugar, and later chapters will look more closely at other dietary influences. Toxicity from mercury (and other heavy metals) has also been outlined. Other factors include:

- Age, because as we get older, immune function declines and yeast takes advantage.
- Serious illness (particularly diabetes, cancer/leukaemia, asthma (because of the treatment) and autoimmune-related diseases), where the illness itself may be associated with a declining immune efficiency (cancer, for example), or the medication used may encourage yeast to spread (steroids such as cortisone, or antibiotics).
- Use of catheters after surgical procedures or trauma, which offer yeasts easy access to the bloodstream unless hygiene is scrupulous.
- Use of inhalant medications for asthma, for example, as these usually contain steroids, which lower resistance to fungal spread.
- Following radiotherapy, as this severely lowers immune efficiency in the tissues affected.
- Low levels of stomach acids (achlorhydria), which encourages both bacterial and yeast colonization of areas where the acids would normally prevent them from going.
- Pregnancy, because of hormonal changes.
- Use of the contraceptive pill or hormone replacement therapy since these, by definition, are hormonal and alter the ecology of parts of the body, allowing Candida to spread.

- Anything which reduces the efficiency of the intestinal flora to control Candida, including prolonged stress and a diet high in fat and/or sugar and alcohol.

Denture hygiene and yeast

A further hazard related to candidiasis was discovered in a study which looked at 50 consecutive patients with respiratory disease who had all developed candidiasis in the mouth and pharynx. It was found that dentures were worn by 32 of the 50 patients and this was thought to be a major predisposing factor in the onset of Candida (among other factors encouraging Candida activity such as the use of cortisone, antibiotics and immune-suppressing sedatives). The researchers said, 'Dentures cause tissue trauma, provide sites for [yeast] colonization and diminish salivary flow. Saliva is necessary for normal oral immune defence.'[11]

It was found that when dentures were treated with antifungal chemicals, this helped to prevent this hazard. Regular sterilization of dentures is suggested as a safe preventative measure along with regular oral rinsing with dilute Aloe vera juice or tea tree oil (antifungal substances; *see Chapter 5*).

Yeast control objectives

Our ultimate attempt to neutralize and control the spread and effects of Candida (for we can seldom get rid of it completely) depends on the use of whatever safe methods we have at our disposal to remove the causes of its spread (see above) and to deprive it of its ideal nutrients while, at the same time, building up and enhancing weakened immune function. The immune system should then be able to get on with the job of keeping Candida in check by itself.

It is this double thrust of activity which must be undertaken if we are to do more than temporarily suppress Candida. The use of antifungal drugs (such as nystatin) can, it is true, destroy a great deal of Candida's potency, and reduce symptoms resulting from its presence and activities in the body. However, the yeast activity will start again soon after the drug is stopped, especially if other changes (such as a reduced sugar intake) are not being made.

Anti-Candida protocol summary

The answer to controlling Candida in the long term (apart from reducing or removing controllable opportunities as discussed above) lies in a multipronged attack to simultaneously:

- deprive the yeast of its optimum nutrient environment ('starve the yeast'), especially sugar-rich foods
- actively kill yeast, using safe, non-toxic methods (and sometimes standard antifungal medication, if the other aspects of the programme are carefully followed)
- actively focus on restoring the body's normal controls over yeast by supporting the immune system and encouraging a healthy intestinal flora ('friendly bacteria')
- help to restore damaged tissues, such as the mucous membrane of the digestive tract (easing 'leaky gut' symptoms)
- support the body's detoxification systems and organs (such as the liver) because toxic debris from dying yeast needs to be eliminated.

As we will see, there are other methods which, it is thought, can help by altering the ability of the yeast to multiply. We will consider these natural, safe alternatives to the use of drugs later.

What about antifungal drugs?

It must, however, be stated that there are conditions in which the use of antifungal drugs[12,13] can be useful, especially if the condition suggests that the process of recovery will be a very long one. In the main, however, once we learn to recognize the symptoms that indicate Candida might be getting out of hand, the natural, non-drug methods described in this book will work, and work well.

The following modern drugs are all used effectively against various Candida infections, depending on where the infection is primarily located (for instance, urinary tract, vagina, skin or systemic): fluconazole (Diflucan), itraconazole (Sporanox), ketoconazole (Nizoral), miconazole (Daktarin, Femeron), amphotericin B (Fungilin), flucytosine (Alcobon).

Side-effects: These are minimal with many of these drugs, especially if only a single dose is prescribed (which is often the case with medications such as fluconazole). The more severe reactions listed below should be seen in context as the medication would commonly be used only in cases of severe systemic candidiasis, where the person is already very ill. When the use of antifungal drugs is prolonged or repeated, the chances of side-effects increase, including:

1 nausea, headache and stomach discomfort (fluconazole, itraconazole)

2 liver dysfunction (ketoconazole, although rarely)

3 severe pruritus (itching), gastrointestinal symptoms,
   fever (miconazole, especially at high doses)

4 fever, headache, backache, vomiting, thrombophlebitis
   and, in some cases, irreversible kidney damage
   (amphotericin B)

5 nausea, vomiting, diarrhoea and (rarely) fatal liver
   disease (flucytosine).

Nystatin is one of the main antifungals used before the
availability of the modern drugs listed above. Nystatin, like
amphotericin B (see above) is derived from fermentation of
a fungus (*Streptomyces albulus* or *S. noursei*). Nystatin is
considered relatively safe and non-toxic, although Truss
and others report that, once it is stopped, when Candida is
apparently under control, a rebound of yeast activity can be
anticipated unless a broad anti-Candida programme has
been adopted.

Nystatin is effective against certain Candida strains
while others are resistant. Not being a broad-spectrum antifungal agent, it allows proliferation of yeasts, such as
Trichophyton, that are resistant to it while Candida is
attacked. This can lead to opportunistic overgrowth of
these resistant yeasts even though Candida is controlled for
the short-term.[14]

A variety of alternatives are discussed in Chapter 5.

The unfortunate aspect of most antifungal drug treatment
is that they are seldom used together with a comprehensive
antifungal dietary and supplement approach, which would
encourage a healthier digestive tract and immune system.

Drugs are seldom necessary at all unless the infection is
severe and widespread since the methods outlined in later
chapters are safer and of proven efficacy.

A reminder

Let us not lose sight of the fact that Candida lives in every one of us and usually produces no symptoms unless the environment in which it lives (our body) has been compromised.

Diagnosis of yeast involvement in health problems is not a case of establishing whether or not yeast is present – because it always is to some extent. Rather, it is the task of the healthcare provider to advise anyone with yeast-related problems to attempt to discover what underlying factors have allowed yeast to proliferate and to focus attention on these – as well as control fungal activity.

Any approach which targets the yeast alone will result in a return of symptoms sooner rather than later. It is not just the yeasts that need to be controlled, but the causes which have allowed them to opportunistically explode into action.

In Chapter 3, we will consider just what can happen to weaken your wonderful defence mechanisms as well as additional ways in which Candida is sometimes allowed to go on the rampage, and so begin to infest other areas of your body.

REFERENCES

1 Edwards J. *Candida Adherence Mycology Research*, Harbor–UCLA Medical Center, Montana State University, 2002
2 Williams R. *Biochemical Individuality*, University of Texas Press, 1979
3 Truss C. *The Missing Diagnosis*, Birmingham, AL: Self-published, 1980
4 Stein J (ed). *Internal Medicine*, London: Little Brown, 1983
5 Odds F. *Candida and Candidosis*, London: Balliere-Tindall, 1988

6 Epstein J. 'Quantative relationships between *Candida albicans* in saliva and the clinical status of human subjects', *J Clin Microbiol* 1980; 12: 475–6

7 Cohen R. 'Fungal flora of the normal human small intestine', *N Engl J Med* 1969; 280: 638–41

8 Truss CO. *J Orthomolec Psychiatry* 1984; 13(2): 66–93

9 Goldberg B. *Chronic Fatigue, Fibromyalgia & Environmental Illness*, Tiburon, CA: Future Medicine, 1998

10 Manning BR. *How Safe are Mercury Fillings?* Los Angeles, CA: Cancer Control Society, 1984

11 Thompson P. 'Assessment of oral candidiasis', *BMJ* 1986; vol 292

12 O'Grady F *et al. Antibiotics and Chemotherapy*, 7th edn, New York: Churchill Livingstone, 1997

13 Bennett J. 'A randomized trial comparing fluconazole with amphoterecin B for treatment of candidemia', *N Engl J Med* 1994; 331: 1325–30

14 Da Prato R. 'Fatty acid ion exchange complexes in treatment of Candida albicans', Concord, CA: report by Arteria Co., 1985

3 | *How Candida gets out of hand*

There are a number of predisposing factors which allow Candida to get wildly out of control. To a greater or lesser extent, these same factors may be involved in the more subtle spread of Candida, which is what happens in the majority of people affected by the symptoms described in Chapter 1.

Anyone affected by a yeast overgrowth is likely to be able to identify a number of interacting 'causes'. Seldom will only one factor be involved. Among the main ones are the following three.

1 An underlying predisposition (a genetic tendency) in some individuals seems to be related to blood type and secretor status. As mentioned in Chapter 1, those who are non-secretors of their blood type are much more likely to be carriers of Candida and to have problems with persistent infections. Blood group O, who are also non-secretors, are the most affected of all. Candida appears to find it easier to colonize (attach to) blood type O cells. In one study, the proportion of non-secretors among patients with chronic candidiasis was 68 per cent.[1]

   One of the protections against Candida which being a secretor offers is the ability to retard/inhibit the ability of bacteria and yeasts, such as *Candida albicans*, to adhere to the surface of mucous membranes.[2] Non-secretor saliva not only fails to prevent attachment of Candida, but may actually promote the binding of Candida to tissues. Women with recurrent vulvovaginal candidiasis (thrush) are much more likely to be non-secretors.[3]

2 Among the major causes of the internal ecological disturbances which lead to Candida overgrowth are the effects of steroids (hormones) in food (residues found in factory-farmed meat and poultry, for example) or in medications (such as cortisone, the contraceptive pill and antibiotics) as well as the long-term effects of antibiotics used as medication or found in factory-farmed animals or their products, such as milk.

Antibiotics and hormones are fed to animals to speed their growth and control the heightened susceptibility to disease that their unnatural lives generate. Anyone who regularly consumes beef, pork, veal and chicken (and many people eat one or more of these daily) will have absorbed prodigious amounts of antibiotic and hormone residues (unless the source of the meat was from a farm that does not use such drugs). Unfortunately, antibiotic residues also find their way into dairy produce (including eggs) unless it is of guaranteed organic origin, so even vegetarians are likely to be affected by antibiotics in food. Low-level intake of these substances over many years may have a devastating effect on the ability to control Candida, as would the regular use of these drugs in the form of medications. This area is yet to be adequately researched, but it does provide one more argument in favour of adopting a near-vegetarian diet that is low in dairy products.

A report in the London newspaper *Daily Telegraph* (19 August 1999) entitled 'Antibiotics, how the cure became a killer', states: 'Eating food containing antibiotic residues exposes humans to a constant low level of [these] drugs.' This not only leads to organisms (bacteria, yeasts) which have become resistant to the medication through constant exposure, but to the likelihood of chronic low-grade infection or overgrowth in those who consume such foods. A study in Holland showed that 14 per cent of the human population in an intensive-farming area were carriers of antibiotic-resistant bacteria.[4]

Yeast infection is also almost certainly rampant in such individuals. Choosing organic sources of food would help to avoid this danger although, unfortunately, agricultural practices which use high levels of antibiotics and steroids on animal and fruit production also leads to run-off of water and effluent containing these medications into rivers, and often into our tap-water supply.[5]

As for avoiding antibiotics as medication, this is not always possible although, in my book *Natural Alternatives to Antibiotics* (Thorsons, 2001), I have explained how it is often possible with the use of a variety of safe alternatives. If antibiotics were used only when absolutely necessary, we would be able to avoid the increasing threat of 'superbugs' which have become resistant to them, largely because of excessive and inappropriate use. And we would also dramatically reduce the spread of the Candida epidemic.[6]

It has also been noted that, because of the hormonal changes that take place during pregnancy, a degree of control over Candida is lost. Yeast, therefore, finds this a good time to expand its activities.

3 Blood sugar imbalances, such as diabetes and hypoglycaemia (low blood sugar), are another 'cause' of Candida overgrowth. Diabetes is a chronic imbalance involving the way the body metabolizes starches, fats and proteins, leading to higher levels of sugar in the

blood than is safe. The dangers of a diabetic state include a greater risk of heart and kidney disease and, most certainly, of yeast infections because of the higher sugar levels. Many people who are not diabetic have wildly fluctuating blood-sugar levels as a result of a range of factors, including adrenaline-releasing habits (such as smoking, caffeine consumption, alcohol, high stress levels, dietary intake of refined sugars and carbohydrates). The 'anti-Candida' diet (*see Chapter 6*) is suitable for diabetics as well as those whose blood sugar levels are unstable.

The following questionnaires can indicate the *possibility* of 1) a diabetic state or 2) a hypoglycaemic state (low blood sugar, which many experts believe can be a prediabetic state).[7] If your answers suggest the possibility of diabetes, you should consult your GP as soon as possible to check this out. If your answers suggest hypoglycaemia, you should consult a nutritionist and/or a naturopath to sort out the dietary and lifestyle factors that need modification.

Diabetes questionnaire

1 Is there a history of diabetes in your family (particularly insulin-dependent diabetes)?
2 Are you over 40 and overweight?
3 Have you become excessively thirsty for no obvious reason?
4 Do you urinate more frequently than in the past (with no actual bladder infection)?
5 Has your appetite increased without any change in your activity levels?
6 As well as the symptoms described in questions 3, 4 and 5, do you find yourself excessively tired for no obvious reason?

If you answered 'yes' to either of the first two questions and to at least one of the other questions, a check-up is called for to rule out the possibility of early diabetes.

Hypoglycaemia (low blood sugar) questionnaire

1 Do you tend to wake up feeling tired and feel more energetic after breakfast?
2 If a meal is delayed or you skip a meal, would you expect to feel edgy, shaky and/or faint?
3 Do you crave sugar-rich foods?
4 Do you regularly (more than once daily) use tea, coffee, chocolate, cola drinks, alcohol or cigarettes to give you an energy boost?

A 'yes' answer to any of these questions suggests the possibility of low blood sugar. More than one 'yes' strongly suggests this to be the case.

A variety of strategies can be followed to help normalize your blood sugar, including supplementing daily with 200 micrograms (mcg) of chromium (known as glucose tolerance factor), eating a diet rich in protein and complex (unrefined) carbohydrates, avoiding sugar-rich foods and the sort of stimulants listed in question 4, and following a 'grazing' pattern of eating little and often.

If Candida is also a problem (and why would you be reading this if it wasn't?), this change in diet will help, but you will still need to follow the anti-Candida protocols outlined in Chapters 5, 6 and 7. A diet rich in simple sugars literally feeds the yeast, and one of the strategies you need to follow is to starve it (while at the same time doing something to eliminate it, as described in later chapters).

Immune system inefficiency

As we have seen in Chapter 2, part of the body's response to an intruder such as Candida is the production of antibodies to confront the particular antigen (a substance which stimulates an immune system response) that is present in the foreign substance or organism. Candida has many antigens, and the efficiency with which the defensive operation is carried out against any particular one of these antigens can, to some extent, be inborn (genetic). There is a wide variation in the degree of response in any one person to the different Candida antigens, which can lead to a state in which the immune system, unable to counteract and expel the yeast invasion adequately, learns to tolerate it in increasing amounts.

Biochemical and metabolic individuality

Research has demonstrated that we are all biochemically unique.[8] This means that there are wide variations in the particular requirements for any of the more than 40 nutrients we require for survival and health. Many of these individual needs are determined before birth and has led to the *genetotrophic* theory of disease causation. This, put simply, says that, because a person has individual inborn requirements which may vary greatly from the theoretical 'average' or 'normal' amount, there is a good chance that one or another of these needs will not be met by the normal dietary intake. This leads, at best, to a lower degree of function and, at worst, to a deficiency state.

To a large extent, this individual inborn (genetic) factor also applies to our ability to handle one or another of the pathogens, or microorganisms, capable of infecting us. This is certainly the case in our ability to handle Candida adequately. It seems that since infestation by this yeast is virtually universal, we are incapable of totally controlling its presence in our bodies. Yet, some people are better able than others to keep it under control and limit its spread. Thus, other people, even without the added complication of factors such as antibiotics and steroid drugs, become 'tolerant' of spread of the yeast.

The most common areas of spread are the mouth, throat and vaginal areas. If this initially produces a degree of immune system reaction and activity, then we would see manifestations of the condition called thrush. This condition would flare up periodically when, perhaps, there are factors that lower the body's general vitality. Eventually, in many cases, the condition might no longer trigger an acute flare-up, but would remain as a semi-permanent, chronic state. This happens when the body becomes 'tolerant' of the yeast and is no longer able to mount attacks against it. It is also an indication of impaired or deficient immune function. The many factors in our environment which can influence this state include stress factors, nutritional inadequacy and toxic pollution as well as the use of specific drugs which weaken the immune system (see above for discussion of steroid and antibiotic use).

Drugs and immune function

Nowadays, we are all familiar with the concept of tissue and organ transplantation. This involves the use of powerful drugs that are designed to prevent the body of the recipient from rejecting the new, foreign tissue or organ. These are called immunosuppressive drugs because it is their primary task to stop the natural defences from working adequately – in other words, to suppress the immune system. The risk of infection and of other diseases resulting from this is all too familiar to patients who have undergone such treatment.

Other drugs such as steroids (hormones) also have this effect. Steroids are used in a variety of conditions ranging from rheumatic disorders to asthma and hormonal imbalances. The most widespread use of steroids, however, is not for the treatment of disease, but in the form of the contraceptive pill. One of the most devastating effects of the long-term use of this type of medication is on the immune system in general, and on the ability of Candida to proliferate wildly, in particular. (The contraceptive pill is discussed more fully below.)

Immune system nutrient support

There is now a variety of nutrient substances known to be absolutely vital for the adequate functioning of the immune system.[7] These include vitamins and minerals with antioxidant properties. Antioxidants are able to slow down, or stop, a process in which substances known as 'free radicals' can cause tissue damage. The major free-radical 'scavengers' are vitamins C and E (acting in conjunction with the mineral selenium) as well as certain amino acids (parts of the protein chain) such as methionine, cysteine and glutathione (which is itself a combination of three amino acids: cysteine, glutamic acid and glycine).

Vitamin B6 (pyridoxine), zinc, manganese and other important nutrients have, when deficient, been shown to be involved in compromising the immune system.[9, 10]

As already mentioned, it is possible for any of the 40-plus nutrients vital to life to be required in extraordinary amounts by any given individual to meet unique inborn needs. Not only is there an inborn difference under normal life circumstances, but these needs can vary markedly during specific conditions, such as infection, stress or pregnancy, in the same person. This means that any vitamin, mineral or other nutrient is capable of upsetting the chain of complex biochemical interactions required for the immune system to function efficiently. The nutrients mentioned above just happen to have a more dramatic impact than some of the others.

Stress and immune function

Stress, which involves repeated, or constant, states of anxiety – and all that this entails in terms of depletion of vital nutrient reserves as well as imbalances of internal secretions and functions – is a major cause of immune incompetence. A new scientific discipline called psychoneuroimmunology studies the direct connection between our emotions and how efficiently, or otherwise, our immune system behaves. The evidence shows a clear link between the mind and the body operating through the defence system, which is meant to protect both. A dramatic demonstration of this connection is the fact that, during periods of stress (students during exam time, for example), people become far more prone to infection. This is an indication of the reduced efficiency of their immune system as well as the increased utilization by the body of vital nutrients, such as zinc and vitamin C, at such times.

The interaction between anxiety/stress conditions and nutritional imbalances leads to the immune system being unable to operate efficiently. If, at the same time, there is an increased demand on the immune system to function efficiently to counteract environmental or nutritional toxicity (air pollution, cigarette smoke, alcohol, caffeine-rich drinks such as coffee, chocolate and tea), then a complex picture emerges in which excess demands, inadequate nutrition (with associated deficiencies) and perhaps drug use, such as the contraceptive pill, will all interact to deplete immune function even further. Let us examine the manner in which commonly used drugs can further complicate the situation.

Antibiotics, the Pill and steroids

It is clear from years of research that the use of antibiotics removes the biological controls over the yeast that lives inside us. As has already been mentioned, a prime site for this to take place in is within the long, dark, warm and moist (ideal environment for yeast) digestive tract which, it should be noted, is also inhabited by upwards of 2.3 kg (5 lb) in weight of other microorganisms, most of which are 'friendly' and helpful to the body.

One such friend is *Lactobacillus acidophilus*, which helps to keep a check on the spread of yeast. When antibiotics are used to destroy pathogenic (harmful) microorganisms which may be causing harm to the body (as in treating an infection), the friendly bacteria in the bowel are also destroyed or severely damaged. When this occurs, yeast, which is totally unaffected by the antibiotic (not being a bacteria), is able to find room for expansion. This becomes even more likely since the resistance of the immune system will be compromised at that time. A similar thing happens with the use of steroid drugs such as cortisone (including cortisone ointments, so commonly prescribed for skin problems, which can cause a yeast increase by being absorbed into the bloodstream). All steroids, including those used in the contraceptive pill, will have a depressing effect on the immune system.

Twenty-first-century woman

Most people with Candida problems are women, and most are under 50 years of age. Why should this be so?

Imagine a young woman who has grown up in an era characterized by the common use of antibiotics and steroid medications. She has had antibiotics prescribed to her over the years for minor problems such as tonsillitis and ear infections. She may then have developed cystitis from time to time and would have taken a broad-spectrum antibiotic for this. She may have suffered from acne which, again, would most likely have been attacked with antibiotics. She may have had steroids for asthma or some other condition. Going on the Pill, and subsequently coming off it and becoming pregnant, would have enhanced the chances of yeast spreading and causing further problems (acne and cystitis are frequent examples of Candida activity). The child in her womb would be exposed to a variety of antigens from all the Candida activity in her body while possibly inheriting a weak immune system (though not all children inherit a weak response). Thus, the pattern will be set to repeat itself.

We have still left out of this picture all the other variables so common in modern society, such as nutritional imbalances, pollution, excessive use of sugar-rich foods (which yeast loves) and stress factors in general. The resulting picture is of a person who is doing just about everything possible to bring about the ideal conditions for yeast to thrive. The result for the general population of such an all-too-typical scenario has been an explosion of Candida-caused problems over the past 40 years or so, which is now reaching epidemic proportions.

An important aspect of Candida's spread is the diet of the individual (covered later) which not only helps to create a less efficient immune system, but actually includes nutrients that support Candida growth. The two main culprits are sugar-rich foods, which all yeasts love, and foods that are themselves associated with yeasts or fungi. In the meantime, it should be evident that many aspects of life in 'civilized' societies are working to the disadvantage of our body's defensive ability and to the advantage of its prospective enemies, such as Candida.

Dr C. Orian Truss' views

Dr Truss, who has done so much to research and publicize the Candida problem, is scathing in his attack of certain drugs which have compounded the problem. Antibiotics are often used inadvisedly in cases where they have no role to play whatsoever. Incorrectly diagnosed viral and fungal conditions may be uselessly treated by antibiotics, for example, which increases the likelihood of the condition worsening. The treatment of acne with tetracycline is another major cause of Candida spread, and Truss insists that anyone suffering from Candida problems cannot ever control the condition if he or she continues to take tetracycline. In many cases, acne is the result of Candida infection and will worsen, rather than improve, with such drug treatment.

In the use of the contraceptive hormone, too, Truss sees great harm. As much as 35 per cent of women on the Pill have acute vaginal candidiasis, and there are undoubtedly many others who have less pronounced changes in this regard as their immune competence is gradually compromised by the hormonal onslaught. As Truss points out, 'Chronic yeast vaginitis tends to be at its worst when progesterone levels are high, as in pregnancy and the luteal phase of the menstrual cycle. Therefore, the progesterone component of contraceptive hormones may well be responsible for their effect.'[11]

The association between Candida vaginitis and emotional problems, such as irritability and depression, frequently appears soon after the first use of the contraceptive pill. It is worth reflecting on the fact that the degree of biological individuality which we display in our individual reactions to any harmful factor, such as Candida, must play a large part in deciding just who will, and will not, succumb to a spread of Candida. Since 35 per cent of women do not control vaginal Candida when on the Pill, we must assume that the other 65 per cent do. This highlights the fact that, for many people, there is an inborn genetic weakness in their ability to meet such a challenge (and this may well be reflected in their blood type and secretor status). For others, this will have been acquired via the factors already mentioned here, such as antibiotic use, and an immune system weakened by stress and nutritional deficiencies. The approach to controlling Candida must include methods that deal with both building up the immune system while reducing as many of the factors as possible which assist the yeast in its advance. Among the most important of these is the elimination of the use (unless absolutely vital) of antibiotics, hormone preparations and contraceptive pills as well as altering the diet to avoid feeding the yeast.

Since yeast loves sugar, it is clear that if a person has additional levels of sugar in the bloodstream, as in a diabetic condition, this will fuel the spread of Candida. For this reason, diabetic individuals are more prone than most to Candida problems and so must be even more rigorous in their efforts to control it.

The possible involvement of mercury toxicity in harming the immune system's control of Candida has been mentioned (*see Chapter 2*) and deserves re-emphasis.

Foods that help to spread Candida

Yeast thrives on carbohydrate-rich foods. This means that we must attempt to deprive it of its sustenance by limiting, or cutting out all together, all sugar-rich foods and refined carbohydrates. Details of how to do this are outlined in the nutritional programme (*see Chapter 6*).

Many experts also consider it important that the intake of any foods that contain fermented products, moulds or fungi be limited.[10] Many anti-Candida programmes emphasize this restriction ('no yeast-based or fermented foods!'), but the reasons for such restrictions are not always explained, and are often not logical.

It must be clearly understood that avoiding such foods is necessary *only if the person with a Candida problem has become sensitized – and is therefore allergic or sensitive to – fungus-related substances.*

If not, there is no reason to add yet another restriction to an already complex programme.

IS AVOIDING YEAST-BASED FOODS NECESSARY OR NOT?
A simple food-exclusion period of 10–14 days, during which time all yeast-based foods are eliminated, is a basic method. At this time, a careful 'symptom' score should be kept (*see Chapter 7*), which will set the scene for a definitive experiment. After a period of yeast-food elimination (it takes at least five days for all traces of the excluded food to be cleared by the system), a 'challenge' can be introduced in which small amounts of a yeast-based food (or a fragment of a yeast tablet) are eaten twice in one day, and any reactions observed.

1 Did the symptoms improve when not eating such foods?

2 Did they return when you reintroduced these foods?

A 'yes' answer to either question suggests that you should investigate further and that you would probably benefit from leaving such foods out of your diet for a while.

The foods that are most suspect if yeast is not well tolerated include vinegar, fermented alcoholic beverages (wine, beer), yeast extracts and spreads, mushrooms, blue cheeses and any food with a mould (*see Chapter 6 for a complete list*). Once Candida is under control, unless there is a yeast sensitivity or allergy, there is no reason to maintain this strict prohibition. But the return of classic symptoms of Candida activity, such as abdominal bloating after eating one of the offending foods, will tell you that it is time to return to a period of strict avoidance.

Just as foods containing moulds or fungi are considered undesirable, it may be that symptoms are worse in humid, damp environments that are conducive to mould and fungus spores being present in the atmosphere. Thus, it is important to eliminate from the home any areas of damp (such as on the walls).

If *Candida* overgrowth is influenced genetically, can it be prevented/controlled?

As we have already seen, some people have a tendency to increased Candida activity, possibly because of their blood type and secretor status. If genetics are indeed a factor in the predisposition to Candida activity (blood type O, non-secretor), then controlling it and keeping it under control will require more work than if the genetic makeup was different.

It is important to understand that a genetic tendency can be either reduced or aggravated by your behaviour, lifestyle and environment. Recent research has shown that more than 50 genetic diseases can be successfully treated using high doses of vitamins.[12] Most of these conditions are rare, inborn metabolic diseases. The genetic changes leading to a Candida susceptibilty are not among those listed by this research, but the fact that other genetic problems can be modified suggests that the presence of a 'tendency' should not be taken as a 'life sentence'. It is likely that such a tendency can be modified.

An anti-Candida programme is not forever!

Candida gets out of hand because we allow it to. We may well do so in ignorance, but it is folly to blame the yeast when we have the power to control it, as millions of people have done before. Once you begin to suspect that your many and varied symptoms (*see Chapter 4*) may be the result of Candida activity, it is time to take responsibility for the situation.

Candida will not go away on its own. Its current spree may be the result of any combination of factors which have released it from the body's normally efficient control. To get it back to where it belongs (or at least to where it can do least harm), we must restore our defence capacity to its optimal level, and stop doing those things that are helping the yeast to thrive. It is as simple as that. You can do this by your own efforts – by the reform of your dietary pattern, by the use of particular nutrient substances, and by reducing the overall levels of stress and pollution in your immediate environment.

Once you have put Candida in its place, you can relax your vigilance to the extent of allowing your diet to contain some 'undesirable' substances from time to time, but you should be aware of the factors which allowed Candida to advance in the first place and avoid these as stringently as possible.

The next chapter looks at the sort of problems that Candida can cause when it gets out of control. Be prepared for some surprises.

REFERENCES

1 Lamey P *et al.* 'Chronic hyperplastic candidosis and secretor status', *J Oral Pathol Med* 1991; 20(2): 64–7
2 Ben-Aryeh H *et al.* 'Oral Candida carriage and blood group antigen secretor status', *Mycoses* 1995; 38(9-10): 355–8
3 Chaim W. 'Association of recurrent vaginal candidiasis and secretory ABO and Lewis phenotype', *J Infect Dis* 1997; 176(3): 828–30
4 Irwin A. *Daily Telegraph*, 19 August 1999, p 6
5 Pizzorno J, Murray M, Joiner-Bey H. *The Clinician's Handbook of Natural Medicine*, London: Churchill Livingstone, 2002
6 Spinillo A *et al.* 'Effect of antibiotic use on the prevalence of symptomatic vulvovaginal candidiasis', *Am J Obstet Gynecol* 1999; 180: 14–17
7 Williams R, Deason G. *Proc Natl Acad Sci (USA)* 1983; 5(7): 163
8 Bland J (ed). *Medical Application of Clinical Nutrition*, New Canaan, CN: Keats Publishing, 1986
9 Colgan M. *Your Personal Vitamin Profile*, London: Blond & Briggs, 1983
10 Williams R. *Nutrition Against Disease*, New York: Bantam, 1981
11 Truss C. *The Missing Diagnosis*, Birmingham, AL: Self-published, 1980
12 Ames B *et al.* 'High-dose vitamin therapy stimulates variant enzymes with decreased coenzyme binding affinity (increased Km): relevance to genetic disease and polymorphisms', *Am J Clin Nutr* 2002; 75(4): 616–58

4 | *Candida and its consequences to your health*

The list of conditions in which Candida has been implicated as a major causative factor is very long indeed. There are dozens of health problems that are yeast-related – some are minor, such as dandruff, but many are disabling in their severity.

How widespread are Candida-related health problems?

According to activist author Gill Jacobs,[1] a third of the populations of Western, industrialized countries have illnesses which are linked to Candida, which translates to hundreds of millions of people.

As has already been mentioned, it is necessary to deduce the involvement of Candida from the history of the person – Have antibiotics been used? Is the person on the Pill? Has cortisone or other steroid, such as prednisone, been taken?

According to Pizzorno *et al.*, 'The best method of diagnosis of Candida-related problems is clinical evaluation – knowledge of yeast-related illness, detailed medical history, [and a] patient questionnaire.'[2] In addition, there should be further tests to support the findings established by clinical evaluation. (A questionnaire which can help to establish the likelihood of candidiasis is found on pages 62–4).

49

The range and type of symptoms can give an indication of Candida involvement. As already established, there is no point in asking a microbiology lab to look for the presence of Candida since we know it to be present in virtually all adults and most children within the first few months of life. So, having concluded from the patient's history and symptoms that Candida seems to be involved, the proof of its involvement can be obtained by carrying out an anti-Candida programme to determine whether or not this reduces or eliminates most of the symptoms.

Before considering these symptoms (at least the major ones) one by one, let us look at a list of the sort of conditions that are known to be the possible result of Candida activity (note that ALL of these conditions, apart from thrush, can result from causes other than Candida):

vaginitis
thrush (oral or vaginal)
endometriosis (disorder involving the lining of
    the uterus)
athlete's foot
acne
dandruff
headaches (migraine type)
fatigue
constipation
bloating
allergy
sensitivity to perfumes, fumes, chemical odours and
    tobacco smoke
poor memory, feelings of unreality, irritability, inability
    to concentrate
depression
numbness, tingling and weak muscles
painful muscles
heartburn

abdominal pain
diarrhoea
irritable bowel syndrome (IBS)
premenstrual syndrome (PMS)
recurrent sore throat and nasal congestion
recurrent ear infection
swelling and discomfort in joints
blurred vision.

The diagnosis of a Candida connection becomes more likely if symptoms are aggravated during damp weather (or in damp places), or in an environment with a lot of mould or fungi. If the symptoms are worse after eating sugar-rich or fungus-containing foods, the argument for Candida involvement becomes stronger.

Local Candida symptoms start before general ones

After looking at some of these conditions more closely, we will pull the key information together in the form of a questionnaire, which should enable you to assess the chances of Candida being involved in your health problems. Truss draws a picture of a typical case of chronic Candida infection in his article 'Restoration of immunological competence to *Candida albicans.*'[3]

He states, after pointing to the influence of multiple pregnancies, birth-control pills, antibiotics and cortisone, as well as other factors that depress the immune system:

'The onset of local symptoms of yeast infection, in relation to the use of these drugs, is especially significant and usually precedes the systemic response. Repeated courses of antibiotics and birth-control pills, often punctuated with multiple pregnancies, lead to ever-increasing symptoms of mucosal infections in the vagina and gastrointestinal tract. Accompanying these are manifestations of tissue injury, based on immunological and possibly toxic responses to yeast products released into the systemic circulation. Many infections are secondary to allergic responses of the mucous membranes of the respiratory tract, urethra and bladder, necessitating increasingly frequent antibiotic therapy that simultaneously aggravates, and perpetuates, the underlying cause of the allergic membrane that allowed the infection. Depression is common, often associated with difficulty in memory, reasoning and concentration. These symptoms are especially severe in women, who in addition have great difficulty with the explosive irritability, crying and loss of self-confidence that are so characteristic of abnormal function of the ovarian hormones.'

Women: *The main Candida target*

Truss then points out that accompanying this sad catalogue is what he calls 'poor end-organ response' resulting in acne, loss of libido (disinterest in sex), menstrual bleeding and cramps, and intolerance to foods and chemicals. The most common (but, by no means, only) type of individual with a Candida infection is a woman, aged somewhere between puberty and the menopause, who has been exposed to some or all of the predisposing factors described previously, and who has some or all of the symptoms outlined in Truss' description above. A mixture of unaccountable vaginal and bowel symptoms, ranging from discharge and itching to bloating, discomfort, diarrhoea and/or constipation, as well as an array of mental–emotional symptoms are typical. Classically, such women are labelled neurotic, which must be the crowning insult to an individual who has literally begun to feel her body and mind giving way in all directions.

Digestive tract colonization

The vaginal and intestinal tracts are the most usual areas for Candida to inhabit since they provide the warm, damp environment it enjoys and the nutrients it thrives on. If circumstances allow, Candida has been known to spread along the entire length of the digestive tract, from the anus to the mouth. The tongue may be coated, and there may be yeast deposits on the insides of the cheeks, on the corners of the mouth and on the gums. White spots and a coated tongue are obvious signs, accompanied by soreness and tingling of the gums. When the oesophagus is affected, the result can be symptoms commonly assigned to 'heartburn'; indigestion and an 'acid stomach' are symptoms which can result from Candida activity in the stomach region. If the infestation is prolific in the small or large intestine, then diarrhoea may be the result. This may be chronic and may be accompanied by mucus and/or blood. There may be cramp-like pain ('spastic colon') and colicky pain, often associated with difficulty in passing normal bowel motions. Bloating and distention of the abdomen is a frequent occurrence with Candida, and there may be a variety of abdominal noises as a result. If constipation is indeed a factor, then haemorrhoids are a likely consequence, as is the possibility of rectal discomfort and itching.

What happens when Candida becomes a fungus?

Candida is what is known as a dimorphic organism. This means that it has two separate identities and that the very nature of Candida changes under certain conditions. Its simple yeast form can turn into a 'mycelial fungus'. The yeast form has no root, but its fungal form produces what are called *rhizoids* – long structures similar to roots – which can penetrate through the mucosa (lining) of the tissue in which they are growing. One of the key controls which prevents this change is the abundant presence of the B-vitamin biotin. In good health, biotin is manufactured in the intestines by friendly bacteria (as well as arriving via the diet). After antibiotic treatment (or anything else which upsets the function of *Lactobacillus acidophilus* and *Bifidobacterium bifidum*, the main friendly intestinal flora), these 'good' bacteria may become severely depleted and unable to manufacture biotin. If this happens, control is lifted from the yeast and the aggressive fungal form emerges to begin its onslaught on new territories in the body.

Supplementation with biotin helps to control this change as does restoration of normal gut flora ecology through supplementation of potent, viable strains of *L. acidophilus* and *B. bifidum*.

It should not, however, be thought that it is enough to simply swallow doses of these bacteria in the hope that this will rebalance the situation. Once damage has occurred to the mucous membrane lining of the intestines, the normal flora (such as *L. acidophilus* and *B. bifidum*) will have great difficulty in attaching to such surfaces. These surfaces often require a period of healing after the elimination of yeast, and special strategies to help with this healing are detailed in later chapters.

PERMEABILITY

Controlling yeast and healing the gut wall are therefore important, and usually successful, strategies in the campaign against Candida. Until this control occurs, the change from yeast to fungus allows penetration by the fungal 'roots' of the boundary between the body proper and the self-contained world of the digestive tract. This increased permeability allows substances to enter the bloodstream that would otherwise be kept out by this boundary. As the fungal form of Candida is invasive, it can use this avenue to enter the body proper, something that happens in some cases of advanced candidiasis.

Another major result of increased gut wall permeability is that large molecules from the food eaten, as well as toxic wastes from the Candida infestation, can pass into and circulate via the bloodstream. These large food molecules are frequently the cause of a wide variety of symptoms that are often of an allergic type, and of an overload of the liver, which has the task of detoxifying the bloodstream.

BRAIN ALLERGIES

If these substances reach the brain, there is a risk of the development of what have been termed 'brain allergies'.[4] These can result in a wide variety of mood and personality problems, ranging from depression, irritability and mood swings to conditions which look for all the world like the symptoms of schizophrenia.

Substances which enter the brain and act upon the receptors there to produce mental and personality symptoms are termed *exorphins*.[5] This differentiates them from endorphins, which are substances produced in the body itself and have roles to play in the functioning of many aspects of the biochemistry of life, including pain control. These externally originating substances (proteins from incompletely digested food, for example) slip into the bloodstream through the gates opened by the fungal 'roots' of Candida and cause havoc with whatever tissues they contact. They are identified as 'foreign' by the immune system, which will attempt to neutralize them. If such a process is long continuing – and it can carry on for many years – then this, in itself, becomes a factor contributing to the ultimate depletion of immune function. The immune system is simply overwhelmed by the constant onslaught. The defensive reaction by the immune system to such substances may result in a wide range of so-called allergic symptoms, including asthmatic attacks, nasal and respiratory conditions, skin reactions, feelings of profound exhaustion, palpitations, and muscle and joint aches and swelling.

REPRODUCTIVE ORGAN DYSFUNCTION

The female reproductive organs are a major site for Candida activity. If the urethra is affected, this can lead to cystitis. If for any of a number of reasons the acidity of the region alters, then the relatively harmless yeast form of Candida can change into the fungal form, and become actively invasive and spread to other regions accessible from the vagina. This can lead to inflammatory conditions in the womb (uterus), fallopian tubes and ovaries.

A wide variety of consequences can result, including the tragic possibility of infertility or sterility. Other symptoms related to Candida involvement in this region include frequent urination coupled with a burning sensation as well as a chronic discharge. Premenstrual and menstrual problems, and the whole range of inflammatory and infectious involvements of the reproductive system, such as endometriosis, can also arise.

WHAT ABOUT PMS?

An American hospital study[6] strongly supported a link between premenstrual symptoms and Candida activity. Thirty-two women with severe symptoms of premenstrual syndrome (PMS) and vaginal candidiasis were treated with a diet low in yeast and sugars (*see Chapter 6*) together with antifungal medication. They were compared with an equal number of women with similar problems who did not receive the anti-Candida treatment. All these patients had previously failed to respond to treatment of their PMS using vitamin treatment and psychotherapy.

The results? Two-thirds of the women receiving anti-Candida therapy showed significant PMS relief whereas none of those who did not change their diet improved. This study clearly showed that if PMS and thrush are both present, then dealing with the yeast will often clear the other symptoms as well, thus implicating the yeast's activities in PMS.

Candida, the mind and the emotions

If either mild or major emotional and psychological symptoms occur at the same time as the sort of symptoms described above, this should alert you to the strong possibility of Candida being a part of the cause. Often, the psychological symptoms may be no more than a general feeling of an inability to concentrate accompanied by memory lapses and feelings of lethargy and exhaustion, often leading to a sense of frustration and anxiety. Symptoms may, however, be far more dramatic, as Truss and others have demonstrated. Truss' first articles on the subject discussed the fact that many conditions are named simply because they fit into a pattern that seems similar to another known illness. Indeed, a combination of symptoms which may have no obvious cause is somehow deemed more 'manageable' medically if it is given a label.

Truss initially reported on six cases, two of whom were women who had been repeatedly diagnosed as 'schizophrenic'. Another woman in this original report was diagnosed previously as having 'multiple sclerosis'.

After all six women recovered with anti-Candida treatment, and all were still in good health up to 17 years after recovery, he asked the pertinent question: 'Were two of these women really schizophrenic, or was it just that *Candida albicans* was responsible for brain function so abnormal that highly competent specialists never doubted the diagnosis of schizophrenia?'

He further asked: 'In the third woman, did *Candida albicans* induce neurological abnormalities sufficiently typical of multiple sclerosis that a competent neurologist would mistakenly diagnose the disease?'

He answers by saying that either the treatment dealt with a yeast infection, which can produce symptoms mimicking these diseases (and many others), or that yeast can actually cause the diseases which are labelled with these names. The indication, after many years of work by Truss and others, is that this is not just a case of remission (which is not uncommon in either schizophrenia or multiple sclerosis), but that Candida can induce symptoms similar to those of other illnesses, which may then be wrongly diagnosed and labelled even by competent specialists.

CANDIDA AND CHRONIC FATIGUE SYNDROME (CFS)

Many people with chronic fatigue syndrome (CFS; also known as ME, or myalgic encephalomyelitis, and postviral fatigue syndrome) have yeast overgrowth and, in many instances, it is the major cause of their condition. This fact came to my attention when Sue Finlay followed the anti-Candida advice given in the first edition of this book and discovered the difference it made in her recovery from CFS/ME.[7] In her article in *The Observer* (London), Sue told of how her doctor, at her insistence, had already prescribed nystatin, and that this treatment had taken her from '. . . being confined to bed, hardly able to stand, in tears all day and suicidal' to a point where '. . . the feeling of being poisoned left me, and a little energy returned.'

She then states that after some months of variable, but gradual, improvement: 'I came on the book, *Candida albicans: Could Yeast Be Your Problem?* by Leon Chaitow. I changed my diet radically. I cut out sugars and refined carbohydrates. All bread, mushrooms, tea, alcohol, vinegar, coffee, chocolate were dropped. All these foods feed the yeast [*see note below*]. I used vitamin supplements to enhance my immune system, olive oil and garlic to attack the yeast, and acidophilus powder to replace the Candida with healthy intestinal flora. I ate vegetables, salads, whole cereals and fruit in abundance. At present, I am able to walk nearly half a mile without total collapse. I am beginning to work in the garden a little. I still have to rest every day and be careful not to overdo things and cause a relapse, but I have had eight months of improvement and am steadily reducing the nystatin.'

Sue Finlay has continued to improve and her message is the one I want people with CFS/ME to hear. It is not all in the mind. Chronic fatigue is more likely to cause depression than be caused by it, and is often largely the result of a faulty immune system weakened by Candida.

Note: Only one thing needs correcting in Sue's story. The stopping of yeast-based foods is not because this 'feeds the yeast', but rather because the system of the person thus affected will usually have become sensitized to yeasts, and eating foods based on yeast, or containing moulds, will further irritate and aggravate such a situation. This sensitization has often been shown by researchers to be present in people with candidiasis.[8]

Understanding Candida

It is clear that the ramifications of Candida infection are not yet fully understood, and that much clarification and research remains to be done. In the meantime, since it is not difficult to identify reasons to suspect its possible involvement, it seems reasonable that a Candida-control programme should be adopted in cases where a combination of both a history and symptoms suggest Candida involvement. Where there is a pattern of ill health similar to any of those briefly described above, whatever previous diagnosis has been made, Candida should at least be considered. The treatment is, after all, harmless, and indeed health-promoting.

All in the mind?

Other conditions that are sometimes confused with Candida involvement are frequently labelled 'psychosomatic'. This can be a way for some doctors to avoid having to admit that they cannot find the cause. Calling such conditions 'functional' or 'psychosomatic' may, if repeated, result in the patients beginning to believe that they are not quite mentally balanced. The terms 'neurotic' and 'nervous' are often ascribed to such individuals, with devastating effects on morale and self-esteem. The yeast or fungal cause may remain unsuspected or, if noted as part of the problem (if thrush is a part of the 'psychosomatic' symptom picture, for example), be simply ignored as a minor piece of the puzzle, unworthy of therapeutic effort.

In patients with CFS/ME, this sort of labelling has led to extreme anger, which has been focused into patient self-help efforts and the emergence of insistent demands for a more scientific examination of their condition. Organizations such as Action for ME and Chronic Fatigue, which has done so much in the UK for getting ME to be taken seriously, were, in fact, the result of the frustration of people like Sue Finlay at being told that their health problems were psychologically based.

There is every reason to believe that Candida overgrowth problems are rampant in modern society. It has been let loose by the use of drugs (often employed in good faith to help other health problems) as well as by dietary patterns which are ideal for the health of Candida rather than the host in which the yeast lives. The number and variety of possible health consequences is mind-boggling and deserves the attention of every individual involved in the healing professions.

The alertness of one man, Dr Truss, has brought about the current increase in awareness of the significance of Candida. He may not be totally correct in his ideas, but the results he has so far obtained in thousands of cases, with the range of symptoms already discussed, simply by paying attention to the yeast component of the problem are proof of the validity of this method of treatment.

There are few areas of health more amenable to self-assessment and self-help, and the information provided in subsequent chapters should enable improvement in most cases where Candida is either the main culprit or is part of the cause of symptoms.

The following questionnaires offer you a chance to assess the possibility of Candida being a major part of your current health picture. Most of the symptoms described may be the result of causes other than Candida. If, however, you have more than one of the indications in List 2 as well as some of the lesser symptoms given at the end of the question-naire, then the 'possibility' increases to a 'probability', especially if you can identify a possible causative link with at least one of the factors in List 1.

Candida questionnaires/checklists

Completing these questionnaires will give you clues as to whether Candida is an active agent in your current health status. Although it is not possible to make a diagnosis by these means alone, a strong indication is possible if there are positive answers in all sections of the questionnaire. This information can then be used to assist you in deciding whether to undertake a Candida-control programme.

1 Have you ever taken a course of antibiotics for an infectious condition which lasted for either eight weeks or longer, or for short periods, four or more times in one year?   Yes/No

2 Have you ever taken a course of antibiotics for the treatment of acne for a month or more continuously?   Yes/No

3 Have you ever had a course of steroid treatment such as with prednisone, cortisone or ACTH?   Yes/No

4 Have you ever taken contraceptive medication for a year or more?   Yes/No

5 Have you ever been treated with immunosuppressant drugs?   Yes/No

6 Have you been pregnant more than once?   Yes/No

Total number of Yes answers:

1 Have you in the past experienced (or do you now experience) recurrent or persistent cystitis, vaginitis or prostatitis?   Yes/No

2 Have you a history of endometriosis?   Yes/No

3 Have you had thrush (oral or vaginal) more than once?   Yes/No

4 Have you ever had athlete's foot or a fungal infection of the nails or skin?   Yes/No

5 Are you severely affected by exposure to chemical fumes, perfumes, tobacco smoke and the like?   Yes/No

6 Are your symptoms worse after taking yeasty or sugary foods or drinks?   Yes/No

7 Do you suffer from a variety of sensitivities/
food intolerances and/or allergies?   Yes/No

8 Do you commonly suffer from abdominal
distention, 'bloating', diarrhoea or constipation?

    Yes/No

9 Do you suffer from premenstrual syndrome
(including fluid retention, irritability)?   Yes/No

10 Do you suffer from depression, fatigue,
lethargy, poor memory, feelings of 'unreality'?   Yes/No

11 Do you crave sweet foods, bread or alcohol?   Yes/No

12 Do you suffer from unaccountable muscle
aches, tingling, numbness or burning?   Yes/No

13 Do you suffer from unaccountable aches
and swelling in joints?   Yes/No

14 Do you have vaginal discharge or irritation,
or rectal itching?   Yes/No

15 Do you suffer from impotence or lack of
sexual desire?   Yes/No

Total number of Yes answers:

Do you have a Candida problem?

If you have answered Yes to one or more questions in the first
list, and to two or more in the second list as well as having
more than one of the following signs and symptoms, then
Candida is probably involved in causing your symptoms:

- symptoms usually worse on damp days
- persistent drowsiness
- lack of coordination
- headaches
- mood swings
- loss of balance

- rashes
- mucus in stools
- belching and 'wind'
- bad breath
- dry mouth
- postnasal drip
- nasal itch and/or congestion
- nervous irritability
- dry mouth or throat
- ear sensitivity or fluid in ear
- heartburn and indigestion.

Some life-threatening implications of Candida overgrowth

We have looked at some of the common, sometimes serious – sometimes merely nuisance – results of Candida overgrowth. Be aware, however, that life itself may be threatened by specific combinations of infections which can result when our immune function is low and Candida is active. Before we discuss the research evidence of a dreadful symbiosis between *Staphylococcus aureus* and *Candida albicans* (both of which, incidentally, can be controlled naturally by friendly bacteria such as *L. acidophilus*), we should briefly examine some of the known disease states which *S. aureus* is known to produce.

TOXIC SHOCK SYNDROME (TSS)
This is typically seen in young women (95 per cent of cases). Those affected by TSS begin to notice symptoms on about the fifth day of their period (tampons are usually being used). Symptoms include a widespread rash, fever, watery diarrhoea, vomiting, sore throat, headaches and aching muscles. The skin may begin to peel off, kidney failure may ensue, and

both respiratory and cardiac complications are common. One or two out of every 10 people with TSS die. The cause is rampant infestation with *S. aureus*, with the symptoms being largely the result of toxins produced by the bacteria.

SCALDED SKIN SYNDROME (SSS)

This condition affects infants, young children and immune-suppressed adults, and usually follows spread of *S. aureus* from a primary infection to somewhere else in the body, such as conjunctivitis. SSS is characterized by fever and profound weakness, and a bright-red, very tender skin rash, with large blisters which slough off in sheets, leaving large areas of the body with no skin at all. Even normal-looking skin shears away with light pressure. Complications are related to disruption of the body's temperature control and fluid balance mechanisms. As with TSS, this condition is caused by a toxin secreted by *S. aureus*.

Between 80 and 90 per cent of *S. aureus* infections found in hospital settings are 'super infections' that are resistant to antibiotics. Other conditions associated with *S. aureus* include gastroenteritis, bone and joint infections (osteomyelitis), septic arthritis, pneumonia, meningitis and inflammatory heart disease.

THE CANDIDA CONNECTION WITH TSS AND SSS

In a series of experiments, Dr Eunice Carlson of the University of Michigan established that, when there was a combined infection of *S. aureus* (or *Streptococcus faecalis* or *Serratia marcescens*) and *Candida albicans*, there was an enormous potentiation of the bacterial infection. Says Dr Carlson: 'Although these studies show that Candida has a strong amplifying effect on the virulence of other organisms (*Staphylococcus aureus*, *Streptococcus faecalis*), how this is achieved is a mystery.'[9]

She continues: 'One possibility is that the candidal infection progress causes physical damage to the organ walls which makes them "leaky", allowing other microbes or chemicals (perhaps toxins), or both, to penetrate more easily: it is also possible that Candida directly stimulates the growth of *Staphylococcus aureus*.'

It is not difficult to understand one of Dr Carlson's explanations since we already know of Candida's ability to make tissues 'leaky', as in the digestive tract, when it changes from its yeast state to its aggressive fungal form.

Dr Carlson looks at the almost inexplicable fact that Candida is seldom automatically dealt with by doctors, and gives the example of Candida infection related to wearing dentures: 'This is now believed to be very common and to occur in 60 per cent of all denture wearers. Biopsies of inflamed areas, however, consistently fail to demonstrate tissue invasion [with Candida]. We can speculate that an equivalent infection of the small intestine would be virtually undetectable.'

So because the presence of Candida is not obvious, it is ignored.

One of the most important messages of this book is that we need to presume that Candida is present and active, based on the individual's symptoms and history, and not on expensive, time-consuming tests, which are commonly inconclusive.

Dr Carlson continues: 'Physicians have reported therapeutic cures for a variety of diverse disease conditions using anticandidal drugs. It now appears possible that this fungus may play a key role in many disease conditions, not by its own toxic or invasive growth, but rather by enhancing secondary infection.'

The methods outlined in the following chapters are suitable for preventing the sort of ailments that Candida produces on its own and the disasters which are possible (TSS and SSS, for example) when other infections occur alongside it.

CANDIDA AND CHRONIC DISEASE

As we have seen earlier in this chapter, Dr Truss has reported on patients who, apparently suffering from multiple sclerosis and schizophrenia, recovered their health when Candida was tackled. Other researchers have pointed to additional connections between yeast overgrowth and a variety of serious health problems.

British researcher Sheridan Stock has identified a number of ways in which Candida overgrowth can contribute towards a weakening of adrenal gland function (the gland which produces adrenaline, the 'energy' hormone) as well as thyroid function.[10]

He states: 'The functioning of the thyroid gland is one of the first activities interfered with by Candida, and it has been observed that 90 per cent of Candida victims have low thyroid function.[11] Underactivity of the adrenal and/or thyroid glands can lead to inadequate hormonal secretions (or an inability of the hormones to act normally), resulting in symptoms which can include extreme fatigue, depression, weight gain, dry skin and sensitivity to cold.'

Stock has also linked Candida activity to many children with learning disabilities and hyperactivity. He reports: 'Mothers of hyperactive children often give a history of candidal vaginitis, particularly during pregnancy, and the children have often been exposed to antibiotics early in life. A low income is frequently part of the picture and leads to poor nutrition and a high-sugar diet.'

Almost all people with HIV/AIDS or other immune-compromised conditions have Candida infections. Eileen Stretch, a Canadian physician, reports that unexplained vaginal candidiasis that is resistant to treatment is often the only sign of underlying immune deficiency.[12]

Note: This does not mean that everyone with chronic Candida problems is severely immune-deficient, but only that everyone who is severely immune-deficient is likely to have Candida overgrowth as a major part of their symptom picture.

In the UK, cancer expert Dr Nadia Coates has stated that she does not believe that cancer develops unless there is a yeast overgrowth in the small intestines which then allows absorption through its mucous membranes of toxic wastes.[1]

A wide range of other chronic conditions, including some forms of arthritis, incapacitating migraines, prostatitis, endometriosis, disabling cystitis, extreme chronic fatigue and widespread allergic symptoms can all be caused by Candida activity. Once again, it is necessary to clarify this by saying that these conditions may also be the result of other causes, but that Candida is frequently a major factor.

The questionnaires presented earlier in this chapter can provide strong indications as to whether or not yeast is likely to be a factor in any symptoms you may have. The subsequent chapters will guide you towards controlling it.

REFERENCES

1 Jacobs G. *Candida albicans – A User's Guide to Treatment and Recovery*, London: Optima, 1994
2 Pizzorno J, Murray M, Joiner-Bey H. *The Clinician's Handbook of Natural Medicine*, London: Churchill Livingstone, 2002
3 Truss CO. 'Restoration of immunological competence to *Candida albicans*', *J Orthomolec Psychiatry* 1980; 9(4): 287–301
4 Philpott W, Kalit D. *Brain Allergies*, New Canaan, CN: Keats Publishing, 1980
5 Hemmings W, *Food Antigens in the Gut*, Lancaster Press, 1980
6 *Female Patient*, July 1987
7 Jorgensen B. 'Baker's yeast allergy in candidiasis patients', *J Adv Med* 1994; 7(1): 43–9
8 Finlay S. *The Observer*, 1 June 1986
9 Carlson E. 'Enhancement by Candida of *S. aureus, S. marcescens, S. faecalis* in the establishment of infection', *Infect Immun* 1983; 39: 1

10 Stock S. 'Conquering Candida', *J Alt Complement Med* 1993; June: 24–6

11 Smith L. 'Trouble in the thyroid', *Health News Rev* 1992; 2: 6

12 Stretch E. 'Clinical manifestations of HIV infection in women', *J Naturopath Med* 1992; 3(1): 12–19

5 | Controlling Candida naturally: supplements, prebiotics, probiotics and herbal extracts

After reading the information in the previous chapters and answering the questionnaire, the answer should be apparent. If Candida is a likely suspect as a cause of your present state of health, then it is necessary to prove this by adopting an anti-Candida programme. If such a programme succeeds in making a major beneficial impact upon your health, you will have proved your suspicions.

Dr W. M. Crook calls this a 'therapeutic trial'.[1] It is the only way to be absolutely sure since there is, as yet, no way of proving that Candida is involved in most health conditions through laboratory tests (although, as already discussed in previous chapters, tests can support what the symptoms and health history suggest).

It is understandable that you would want certainty that Candida is the culprit. Certainty is, however, not usually possible. If a searching evaluation of the current symptoms and signs plus a review of past history looks like a 'Candida picture', then the only real choice you have is to either go on as you are or introduce anti-Candida measures.

Pizzorno and his colleagues[2] state this succinctly: 'The best [diagnostic] method: clinical evaluation – knowledge of yeast-related illness, detailed medical history, patient questionnaire.'

If a culture were made of your fluid discharges, tissues or excreta, it would almost certainly display the presence of Candida somewhere in your body. However, this would not prove or disprove anything as far as your symptoms are concerned since a positive test result could also be obtained from almost every adult in the land, with and without symptoms.

Only by looking at the known and suspected pattern of symptoms built up around Candida activity can we make a guess as to its active presence (as opposed to its benign presence, when your immune system and intestinal flora are keeping it under control).

The only real proof to connect Candida with your symptoms lies in the treatment results. If your health improves after controlling Candida, then you will know that what you assumed was accurate and that your anti-Candida programme was the correct one. The very least that you will have achieved is a reformed dietary pattern, and a supplemented intake of some harmless vitamins and other nutrients, as well as building up your immune system's ability to combat its adversaries.

It is reasonable to ask whether it is necessary to attack Candida that is active in a localized region (such as oral or vaginal thrush) by using an approach aimed at the intestinal tract. Years of clinical experience have shown that unless the 'reservoir' of yeast overgrowth in the intestines is controlled, local infections in the vagina are likely to recur. Although not all medical experts agree on this, there appears to be strong evidence that dealing with intestinal yeast is an important part of effectively dealing with vaginal thrush problems.[3]

Researchers writing in the *American Journal of Obstetrics and Gynecology* detailed a study in which they treated women with serious vulvovaginal candidiasis. These women were also assessed for intestinal Candida activity and, in all 258 women in the trial, such activity was evident. The patients were divided into two groups – one received antifungal medication both by mouth (for the intestines) and vaginally, the other received antifungal medication locally for the vagina, but took dummy tablets (as a placebo control). The medication was used for just one week and the women were reassessed after one week, three weeks and seven weeks. The results showed that 88 per cent of those receiving both the digestive tract and local antifungal approach were clear of Candida overgrowth compared with 75 per cent of those who had intravaginal therapy only.[4] While this shows significant, although not massive, benefits when both local (vaginal) and intestinal Candida are treated simultaneously, there is an even more important result when both are attacked: a reduction in recurrence, which was far higher among those women not treated for digestive yeast overgrowth. So, if you treat localized thrush and/or yeast-induced vaginitis without treating the overgrowth in the intestinal tract, you will probably improve, but there will be a greater probability of a recurrence. If the intestinal overgrowth is treated, however, especially if with a comprehensive approach (not just one week of medication, as in the above-described study), recurrence will be far less likely.

Controlling Candida naturally

Achieving control over Candida falls into a number of different aspects:

1 Avoiding those factors which are encouraging yeast overgrowth, including – wherever possible – steroid and antibiotic medications.

2 Use of antifungal products, possibly including caprylic acid, berberine, garlic and oregano oil, as well as nutrients such as biotin, which retards yeast from changing to its fungal form.

3 Starting and sticking to an anti-Candida dietary pattern (described later in this chapter), with avoidance of sugar and refined carbohydrates as an absolute requirement (*see Chapter 6 for the diet in detail*).

4 Improving the health of the intestines especially in relation to permeability (a 'leaky gut') and recolonizing it with friendly bacteria (including the use of prebiotics and probiotics as described below).

5 Improving detoxification functions, specifically those involving the liver.

6 Improving overall immune function through an altered lifestyle and diet, and possibly using vitamin/mineral and herbal supplementation.

The sequence in which the different elements of an anti-Candida programme are introduced can vary, depending on the particular needs of the given individual. For example, sometimes it is necessary to spend some weeks supporting liver function so that it will be better able to handle the detoxification role it plays as yeast dies off. In other instances, the state of the digestive tract requires attention before anything else is attempted. Whatever sequence is adopted, the specific needs of the individual are the deciding factors as to the details of each aspect of the whole programme.

I. AVOID THOSE FACTORS WHICH SUPPORT CANDIDA ACTIVITY

Unless absolutely necessary, the contraceptive pill, hormone replacement, other forms of steroid medication (such as cortisone) and antibiotics should be avoided for the duration of the anti-Candida programme. Dietary strategies which support a healthy intestinal ecology – including healthy friendly bacteria – are described in Chapter 6, but the basic elements of this part of the programme involve avoiding foods which feed the yeast, such as sugar and refined carbohydrates (white-flour products, for example).[5, 6]

Pre- and probiotic strategies are discussed later in this chapter, along with how to encourage healthier friendly-bacteria colonies and the other factors which can damage the ecology of the intestinal tract, including a high-fat intake and high stress levels (which change acid/alkaline levels and so change the environment in which the bacteria live). The healthier your intestinal tract, the less chance Candida has of invading and colonizing the territory.

2. USE ANTIFUNGAL PRODUCTS

Just as different bacterial strains are resistant to particular antibiotics, so different strains of Candida can be more or less susceptible to different herbal products and drugs. Recommended herbal extracts include caprylic acid, garlic, berberine, Kolorex, oregano oil and pau d'arco. Other products are sometimes used, but this selection includes those that I have found most useful over many years of treating chronic candidiasis.

CAUTION: These herbal/plant extracts should not be taken by pregnant or nursing women.

CAPRYLIC ACID, an extract of coconut palm, destroys Candida effectively. It has been used successfully to treat patients with severe intestinal Candida when in a time-release form that allows its release in the lower intestinal tract. If not used in this form, caprylic acid is less effective as it will be absorbed in the upper intestinal region. Caprylic acid mimics the fatty acids produced by normal bowel flora which are a major factor in the body's control over Candida.[7, 8]

Caprylic acid is recommended in preference to commonly used antifungal drugs such as nystatin (discussed later in this chapter), which is itself yeast-based. Research at the Washington University School of Medicine shows that, ultimately, when nystatin treatment is stopped, the result is often even more colonies of yeast developing than were present before its use. Caprylic acid has no such rebound effect when its use ceases after Candida is controlled (we never actually get rid of the yeast, so the goal is only to get it back under control).

Caprylic acid is now widely available in the UK at healthfood stores and some pharmacies. The suggested dosage varies, but good results have been obtained by using 1000–2000 mg time-release capsules three times a day with meals. It is an alternative option to oil of oregano.

UNDECYLENIC ACID/CALCIUM UNDECYLENATE is a safe and useful broad-spectrum antifungal, extracted from castor bean oil. Its action is similar, and usually more potent, than, caprylic acid. Undecylenic acid is a major ingredient of combination formulations that also contain caprylic acid and other antifungal agents such as pau d'arco. To ensure that these fatty acids are delivered to the appropriate part of the digestive tract, it is important to use time-release capsules to avoid their absorption too high up in the gastrointestinal tract.

GARLIC has been the subject of worldwide research.[9] Russian scientists have proved its long-reputed antibacterial activity by introducing garlic extract into colonies of bacteria, which ceased to function within minutes. Fresh garlic juice was used in these tests. Reports in Western medical and scientific journals confirm such claims,[10] in this case, against *Salmonella typhimurium* and *Escherichia coli*, two extremely active microorganisms. Garlic is extremely effective against yeast and fungi,[9, 11, 12] and part of your anti-Candida campaign should include the daily intake of either fresh garlic or garlic in capsule form. The former is preferred, though the latter is an acceptable compromise. Take two to three garlic capsules, morning and evening, after meals or eat as much raw garlic as you can learn to enjoy. Slice it finely on cooked vegetables or crush it onto salads, or simply eat it, clove by clove, with fish or poultry as many Greeks do. The suggested dosage is 400–600 mg three times a day with food (supplements should contain approximately 4000 mcg of allicin per capsule) or one clove of fresh garlic daily.

BERBERINE is derived from the goldenseal (*Hydrastis canadensis*), barberry (*Berberis vulgaris*) and Oregon grape (*Berberis aquifolium*) plants. It has a wide spectrum of antibiotic activity against bacteria, protozoa and fungi. Berberine's action against Candida has been shown to be more powerful than most medical drugs commonly used for these pathogens. In studies, berberine deactivated not only *Candida albicans*, but 10 other fungal species.[13, 14]

Berberine's action against Candida prevents its overgrowth after antibiotic use and also helps to repopulate the gut with friendly bacteria. Berberine is an antidiarrhoea agent with immune-enhancing capabilities while, at the same time, being able to destroy bacteria, yeasts and viruses – a catalogue of benefits.

ECHINACEA ANGUSTIFOLIA (purple coneflower), the Native American herb, offers similar benefits to those of berberine. It is a powerful antiviral and antifungal agent, and an immune-system enhancer. Some products combine *Echinacea*, *Hydrastis* and berberine together with other immune-enhancing nutrients, such as zinc and vitamin C.

Suggested dosages include:
- 1–2 g of dried bark or root of *Berberis vulgaris* or *Hydrastis canadensis* (powdered or as a tea) three times daily

OR

1–1 1/2 teaspoons (4–6 ml) of a tincture of either of these plants (diluted 1:5), three times daily,

OR

1/4–1/2 teaspoon of a fluid extract of either of these plants, three times daily.

The dosage recommendations for encapsulated products is 750–1500 mg daily in divided doses.

HOROPEITO and Mikoplex are the brand names of an extract of the New Zealand plant *Pseudowintera colorata*, formerly known as Kolorex. This very slow-growing shrub has leaves which contain a strong antifungal agent – polygodial – which is particularly effective against *Candida albicans*. Studies at the University of Canterbury in New Zealand found that polygodial compared favourably with the powerful pharmaceutical antifungal amphotericin B.

In one such study, Horopeito/Mikoplex was prescribed to 22 patients (aged between 5 and 45), all of whom had chronic intestinal candidiasis. All patients had been previously treated with antifungal drugs with only short-term benefits. The patients took one capsule of Horopeito/Mikoplex twice daily for two weeks while 10 patients were treated with the antifungal drug Diflucan (fluconazole; 50 mg a day for seven days). Some improvement was seen in patients from both groups within three days, and in all patients taking Diflucan and 15 of those taking Horopeito/Mikoplex within seven days. Twenty of the Horopeito/Mikoplex patients showed marked improvement after two weeks. The researchers said: 'All the patients were repeatedly consulted in a month after the trial: 80 per cent of the patients treated with Diflucan had clinical and bacteriological relapses while only 32 per cent relapsed in the group treated with Horopeito/Mikoplex. No adverse reactions were observed in both groups.'[15]

Further research at the University of California found that Horopeito/Mikoplex was 32 times more effective against *Candida albicans* when combined with the main active extract of the South American spice anise seed (*Pimpinella anisum*). Toxicity has seldom been reported with either herb, although nausea and a headache in the first few days of use may be experienced, probably due to yeast die-off.

The recommended dosage is one capsule containing approximately 350 mg daily of polygodial taken at the same time as 450 mg of anise seed (one capsule of each).[15]

OREGANO OIL. The essential oil of oregano contains powerful antifungal compounds. Side-effects are minimal, however, although allergic reactions to oregano oil can occur. It is advisable to stop taking oregano oil if allergic signs or symptoms appear. This is one of the most useful antifungals and is widely available. If possible, it should be taken in an enteric-coated capsule which delays its release until it reaches the intestinal tract.

The recommended dosage is 0.2–0.4 ml in an enteric-coated capsule twice a day between meals as an alternative to caprylic acid or calcium undecylenate.[16–18]

PAU D'ARCO (also known as taheebo) is the inner bark of a South American tree which has a long history of folk use in the treatment of a wide variety of afflictions. Researchers have shown that pau d'arco extracts (containing lapachol) have strong antifungal actions and are particularly effective against *Candida albicans*. It is commonly taken in the form of a tea, taken several times daily.[19]

ALOE VERA. The juice of this desert plant is a powerful antifungal agent. The healing qualities of *Aloe vera* have been known since Phoenician times. In recent years, attention has been drawn to its usefulness in a range of digestive conditions. Professor Jeffrey Bland has demonstrated that the activity of the fresh juice on Candida can help sufferers. He writes: 'In a study of 10 subjects, six had markedly altered stool cultures in microbiological assays. Four of these had indications of yeast overgrowth in their stools before taking *Aloe vera*, and had reduction in yeast abundance after *Aloe vera* supplementation. *Aloe vera* has an antifungal action as well as improving overall bowel flora condition and improving the local acidity balance . . . It [also] promotes a favourable balance of gastrointestinal symbiotic bacteria.'[20]

Aloe vera juice has a similar effect on bacterial and fungal infections of the skin, and can be applied to such conditions locally. One or two teaspoonfuls of *Aloe vera* juice in water should be taken twice daily by anyone with Candida problems. (*Note:* Once opened, *Aloe vera* juice should be kept refrigerated. The optimum shelf-life after opening is about one month.)

TEA TREE OIL (*Melaleuca alternifolia*) is the remarkable extract of an Australian plant with powerful antifungal properties. Douching daily with a 1 per cent solution in water (or, once a week, soaking a tampon into such a solution and inserting it into the vagina, leaving it there for no more than 24 hours) can be very helpful for vaginitis or cervicitis. This approach is useful whether the cause is Candida or *Trichomonas*. Tea tree oil can also be used as a gargle or mouthwash (one drop in a tumbler of water) for oral thrush, or applied directly onto the skin as an ointment. It is somewhat irritating to the skin if used neat as an oil, but there are many products with a 15 per cent tea tree oil content which are relatively non-irritating). Another use is as a pessary for vaginal thrush.

CHAMOMILE (*Matricaria chamomilla*) contains antifungal substances in its oil extract. Used as a tea or for topical application, it has soothing qualities similar to taheebo (pau d'arco, *see page 78*).

TANNATE PLANT EXTRACTS. Plant extracts called tannates (such as tannin in tea) are powerful antifungal agents. When taken orally, they destroy yeasts selectively, including their spores, without harming the natural flora of the body. There are also formulations for use in the mouth when Candida is locally active and for intravaginal use when thrush is evident. An advantage of using tannates is that they act only in the digestive tract, and are not absorbed at all elsewhere, unlike fatty acids, which may be absorbed too high up in the digestive tract unless delivered in suitable time-release capsules.

Tannates are also useful for detoxifying heavy metals from the body and are, therefore, suitable for use when mercury toxicity, for example, is a factor in immune suppression (*see Chapter 2*).

Up to six (but usually three) capsules of 600 mg each are suggested with every meal for at least two – and ideally up to eight – weeks for chronic candidiasis.

ANTIPARASITIC HERB AND PLANT EXTRACTS. A recent development has been the use of extracts of citrus (usually grapefruit) seeds, which have been promoted as a safe, natural anti-Candida and antiparasitic agent. The evidence for these benefits remains anecdotal, with little research evidence to back up these claims.

Additional antiparasitic herbal assistance is found with berberine (see above) and also *Artemisia annua*, a traditional Chinese herb which is commonly combined with grapefruit seed extract as an antifungal and antiparasitic medicine. This should not be confused with *Artemisia absinthum*, a traditional European herb, which can be toxic and is illegal in some countries.

A number of safe, antiparasitic herbal combinations are available at healthfood stores. Most are effective against both yeasts and parasites, such as combinations of berberine, *Artemisia* and grapefruit seed extract.

BIOTIN is an important nutrient to combat Candida activity which is taken with probiotic supplementation. Research in Japan has indicated a fascinating way in which Candida can be deterred from altering from its relatively harmless yeast form into its invasive and dangerous mycelial (rooted) form.[21] This change occurs more rapidly in a medium that is relatively biotin-deficient. Also called vitamin H, biotin produces a number of skin conditions when in deficiency in humans, including a dermatitis that is characterized by a greyish, dry, flaky appearance. This is accompanied by a lack of appetite, nausea, lassitude and muscle pain. It is interesting to note that all of these symptoms are also commonly seen when Candida is proliferating, and it is worth questioning whether the supposed symptoms of biotin deficiency are not, at least in part, the result of the Candida activity brought about by the deficiency.

Eggwhite contains a substance called avidin, which is capable of combining with biotin, thus neutralizing its usefulness in the body. For this reason, raw egg should not be included in the anti-Candida diet (as avidin is destroyed by cooking).

Biotin should be taken as a supplement three times daily (between meals) in doses of 350–500 mcg in association with *Lactobacillus acidophilus*.

OLIVE OIL (oleic acid) is a further aid in the prevention of the transformation of Candida to its mycelial form. Olive oil contains a substance called oleic acid, which acts upon the yeast in a similar way to biotin. The recommended amount of olive oil is six teaspoons daily, divided into three doses. This can be included in the meal (added to salad or cooked vegetables), or taken before or after meals as desired. Ensure that the olive oil is virgin, cold-pressed and organic, if possible.

3. THE ANTI-CANDIDA DIET

This represents the single most important aspect of the entire programme (*see Chapter 6 for the detailed diet*). Over the nearly 20 years since the first publication of this book that I have been actively teaching people how to follow an anti-Candida diet, a significant number of patients have informed me that they benefited enormously from the change of diet alone when, for one reason or another (such as economic factors or a lack of availability of specific products), they did not follow the entire programme. Depriving yeast of its main food source, sugar, is far and away the most important (and for some people, the most difficult) part of an anti-Candida approach.

4. HEALING THE INTESTINES, REDUCING PERMEABILITY AND REPOPULATING WITH FRIENDLY BACTERIA

For friendly bacteria to rapidly recolonize the territory taken from them by Candida (or other bacteria or yeasts), a number of elements need to be in place: an improved environment, including the right sort of food for these bacteria ('prebiotics'); deactivation of the yeast (as described in the previous section); healing of the irritated, often inflamed and undesirably permeable mucous membranes to which they need to attach; and a plentiful supply of colonizing organisms. Researchers[22] suggest that a combination of pre- and probiotics (known as symbiotics) is the ideal approach, and that is what is recommended in this programme.

Prebiotics

The way in which the normal flora of the large intestine (bifidobacteria) are nourished has a dramatic effect on how well these bacteria function. Since they perform a number of important functions, including manufacturing certain vitamins and detoxifying the intestines as well as controlling undesirable bacteria and yeasts from spreading, it is in our best interests to keep them healthy. The functional efficiency of the bifidobacteria is reduced when the diet is rich in animal fats and refined carbohydrates. On the other hand, certain foods – known as prebiotics – can improve their function.

A prebiotic has been defined as a 'non-digestible food ingredient that beneficially affects the host by selectively stimulating the growth and/or activity of one or a limited number of bacteria in the colon, and thus improves host health'. The beauty of prebiotics is that they specifically help only the friendly bacteria while not nourishing disease-causing organisms; also, despite being carbohydrate-based, prebiotics are not digested and absorbed and, therefore, do not increase your weight.

Among the best known of the prebiotics are fructo-oligosaccharides (FOS), gluco-oligosaccharides (GOS) and lactosucrose, which have all been shown to be capable of improving the status of the intestinal flora (bifidobacteria and *L. acidophilus*) after only a short period of time.

Many fruit and vegetables contain prebiotics such as FOS, including onion, garlic, banana, asparagus, leek and Jerusalem artichoke. To ensure an intake of prebiotics sufficient to make a difference to the bowel ecology, a great deal of such food needs to be eaten, so supplementing with powdered forms of FOS, for example, is suggested to boost intake.[22, 23]

An additional boost to the efficient functioning of bifidobacteria and *L. acidophilus* is the presence in the intestine of a non-resident organism, *Lactobacillus bulgaricus*, one of the yoghurt-making bacteria, together with *Thermophilus*. Thus, supplementation with *L. bulgaricus* will have a prebiotic, or bifidogenic, effect in supporting the function of the normal flora. Research shows that not less than 4 g, and ideally 8 g of FOS (available from most health-food stores) should be taken daily to help your friendly bacteria.

Probiotics

When antibiotics or steroid medications are used, they inevitably destroy a number of the 'friendly' bacteria that inhabit our digestive tract which, as well as providing other valuable symbiotic (mutually beneficial) contributions to the body, also act as a controlling element to stop Candida (and other undesirable yeasts and bacteria) from spreading.

In the average bowel, there are *huge* colonies of micro-organisms which can weigh, in total, 1.5–2 kg (3–5 lb). In number, the friendly flora of the bowel exceed the total number of cells in your body. Certainly, they are not all helpful or friendly but, when you are healthy, most are. To repopulate the bowel with the more helpful residents requires large quantities of these friendly varieties – mainly, *Bifidobacterium* and *Lactobacillus acidophilus*, which lives mainly in the small intestine. When these are recolonized, intruders such as Candida are pushed back and often eliminated from the area.

Dr Khem Shehani, a leading researcher into probiotics and their medicinal properties (therapeutic use of friendly bacteria), is quite clear on the usefulness of lactobacilli against yeast infections: 'Continuing research has revealed that supplementing the diet with friendly bacteria, like *acidophilus* and other compatible organisms such as *Bifidobacterium bifidum* . . . should help in curing candidiasis.'[24]

This viewpoint is confirmed by Japanese research,[25] which has examined the degree of overgrowth of Candida as ascertained by the levels found in the faeces of leukaemia patients receiving drug therapy. Their Candida counts were very high before treatment with bifidobacteria supplementation, which reduced levels of Candida in the faeces of some patients from a high of 10,000,000 per gram to a mere 10,000 per gram after treatment. The effectiveness of bifidobacteria in achieving this was seen in all 16 patients treated whereas 11 'control' patients, who did not receive

Bifidobacterium supplementation, showed no change at all in their Candida levels.

Many researchers report that *Lactobacillus acidophilus* and *Bifidobacterium* actually manufacture substances which retard the growth of Candida, and this is borne out when *L. acidophilus* is added to culture dishes in which Candida is growing, where its ability to slow and even stop its growth is evident.

An additional bonus is received when bifidobacteria are supplemented against Candida, as these probiotics have a uniquely powerful ability to enhance detoxification through the liver as well as detoxifying the intestinal tract itself.

For these reasons, it is worth sharing the words of leading American nutrition expert Dr Jeffrey Bland:[26]

'We have been very excited about an alternative therapy for the management of Candida infection which avoids the use of anti-yeast medication (such as nystatin). It is well recognized that a disturbed flora of the GI [gastrointestinal] tract can establish a proper environment for yeast proliferation. By reinoculating [supplementing] the bowel with the proper symbiotic acid-producing bacteria – *Lactobacillus acidophilus* and bifidobacteria – there is a reduction in the compatibility of the intestinal environment for the yeast proliferation. We have recently used an oral supplement of *Lactobacillus acidophilus* – this has been extremely successful in reducing *Candida albicans* in the intestinal tract. The *Lactobacillus acidophilus* is given as a dry culture.'

This approach of using friendly bacteria to repopulate the digestive tract plays a major part in the strategy outlined in this chapter, and is suitable for anyone with active Candida overgrowth. These friendly bacteria (*L. acidophilus* and *Bifidobacterium*) are among the first of the anti-Candida supplements you should introduce, together with live, cultured yoghurt and/or sour milk with meals (provided you are not allergic to dairy products). These two major probiotic 'bacterial friends' will help to control yeast which may have filled the vacant space left behind in the aftermath of antibiotic use (or other factors, such as an imbalanced high-sugar/high-fat diet).

Bacterial cultures intended for supplementation are available in a number of forms, such as powders or in capsules. Cultured milk products (such as live yoghurt) containing *L. acidophilus* and *B. bifidum* organisms can also play a part in the anti-Candida programme, although the numbers present in such products are relatively low compared with the high-potency powders and capsules currently available.

Essential probiotic knowledge [27]

When lactobacilli or bifidobacteria are supplemented, it is vital to ensure that the product you are taking contains not less than one billion viable, active (potentially colony-forming) organisms per gram. This almost always means that the product will need to be kept refrigerated once it has been opened, and cool at all times. The potency (number of organisms per gram) needs to be guaranteed at the time of purchase – not at the time of manufacture.

When taking these two organisms therapeutically – as in an anti-Candida programme – they should be taken in equal quantities in water. The amount taken will vary with your condition, but is usually around 5–10 g a day of each in divided doses between meals for a week or more, followed by half that quantity for the duration of the programme, which usually runs for three to six months, depending on your progress. A lower 'maintenance' dose is commonly suggested for long-term use.

A rough guide is that a teaspoonful of powdered probiotic culture is equal to about 2 g, which – depending on potency – equals around two to three billion organisms of each type per teaspoonful.

Powders are usually taken two to three times daily between meals whereas encapsulated products are usually taken with meals. A supplement of *Lactobacillus bulgaricus* is also often suggested, in powder form at a dose of around a teaspoonful of powdered culture with each meal, as an immune-enhancing strategy as well as to improve the colonizing ability of *L. acidophilus* and *B. bifidum*.

Children under the age of seven should be supplemented with *Bifidobacterium infantis* and *not* the adult version, and not with *L. acidophilus* unless there has been a recent infection or use of antibiotics – in which case, they should be supplemented with both in a ratio of 50:50.

A child weighing 35 kg (77 lb or 5 1/2 stone) should take half the adult quantity of probiotic organisms, and one weighing 20 kg (44 lb or 3 stone) or less, a quarter of the adult dose.

Precautions when supplementing with probiotics
It is suggested that probiotic products containing additional organisms other than *L. acidophilus*, *Bifidobacterium* or *L. bulgaricus*, such as *Streptococcus faecium* and *Lactobacillus casei*, should be avoided. This is because the only reason to include these in any mixture is usually a commercial one; there are few dangers – except for a loss of quality and a waste of money.

You should also make sure that the container in which the organisms are purchased is made of dark glass and that there is a guarantee of potency up to an expiry date on the label, and that refrigeration is recommended.

Avoid liquid probiotic products – stick with powders (best) or capsules. Avoid tablets, as the process of manufacture destroys much of the potential of the organisms to colonize.

If possible, ensure (by asking the retailer or manufacturer) that the product was not centrifuged – a process whereby the organisms are separated from the supernatant (the 'soup' in which they are grown) which is damaging to them and reduces their colonizing potential.

Try to obtain specific strains of the organisms, for example, LB-51, a superefficient strain of *L. bulgaricus*, and DDS-1, a well-documented superstrain of *L. acidophilus*.

If you are dairy-sensitive, make sure that the culture was not grown on a dairy base. Many other options are available from the better manufacturers.

Wherever possible, obtain each organism in a separate container as they are not compatible with each other when kept together, even if freeze-dried. An exception to this is when the *L. acidophilus* and *Bifidobacterium* have been separated by a special process of microencapsulation.

Follow the manufacturer's advice regarding when the product should be taken (at mealtimes or away from food).

Do not be confused by claims that particular products are 'human strains' or 'human compatible'. All high-quality probiotic products are suitable for human use.

If you ask the questions suggested here, you will obtain products of a quality appropriate for an anti-Candida programme.

Many practitioners suggest waiting for a week or two after commencing an anti-Candida programme before probiotic supplementation. I prefer to start them immediately as they enhance detoxification of the waste products of the yeast, which is dying off, and the sooner recolonization can start, the better. If the gut wall has become inflamed due to Candida activity, then recolonization may take longer than is ideal. However, the strategies suggested below can assist in this.

The products I usually recommend, based on their use by thousands of patients for over 15 years of experience, are those manufactured by Natren, who usually recommends that their products be taken away from meal times (an hour before, ideally), and BioCare, who usually suggests that their products be taken with meals, as well as Culturelle, a probiotic product made by US manufacturer CAG Functional Foods. This does not mean that there is no value in other products, only that these are my preferences.

Healing the intestinal mucous membrane
At the same time that prebiotic and probiotic supplementation commences, particular attention should be given to ensuring that the intestinal walls are in a state that will allow recolonization by the friendly bacteria. If Candida overgrowth has caused damage to the walls of the intestinal tract, then recolonization will be difficult. There are other dangers as well. UK expert Sheridan Stock states: 'Candida damages the intestinal mucosa which leads to an increase in the permeability ('leaky gut' syndrome) which allows large molecules of incompletely digested food protein (and yeast byproducts) to enter the bloodstream, thus provoking immune responses.'[28]

Food intolerances and allergies play a large part in the symptoms experienced by many people suffering Candida overgrowth, and healing the 'leaky gut' is a key element in eliminating these symptoms.

Conditions which are known to be associated with a leaky gut include asthma, ankylosing spondylitis, Crohn's disease, eczema, food allergy, irritable bowel (IBS), inflammatory joint disease, malabsorption, psoriasis, Reiter's disease, rheumatoid arthritis, schizophrenia and ulcerative colitis.[29, 30]

So, to allow better attachment for the friendly bacteria as well as reducing the load on the immune system, attention to irritated intestinal mucous membranes is important. Fortunately, there are a number of natural products which can assist in normalizing this damage. These are best used under expert guidance, however – not for reasons of risk, but to ensure that what is being done is the appropriate course of action.

Among the products which may be used are:

1 L-Glutamine, an amino acid which enhances recovery of damaged mucous membranes
2 *N*-Acetyl-glucosamine (NAG), an amino sugar which is a raw material for reconstruction of tissue damage, and which also both assists recolonization by friendly bacteria and retards Candida's ability to 'stick' to the wall of the intestines
3 Rice-bran oil (gamma-oryzanol), a superbly soothing substance which helps in tissue recovery
4 Butyric acid, a normal product of the friendly bacteria, also found in olive oil, which helps in mucous membrane healing
5 FOS (fructo-oligosaccharides, already discussed in this chapter), usually extracted from vegetables such as Jerusalem artichokes. FOS encourages healing of the gut wall and recolonization of friendly bacteria.

These substances may be prescribed individually or in various combination products available from healthfood stores.

Additional assistance to the digestive process is often needed, provided by the addition to the supplement list of enzyme complexes and by methods for helping to ensure that adequate digestive acids are present in the stomach during digestion. This might call for supplementation with hydrochloric acid capsules or, preferably, with herbs which promote the natural production of acids (such as 'Swedish bitters'; *see Chapter 6*).

5. DETOXIFICATION AND LIVER SUPPORT

Toxicity in the intestines is associated with an unhealthy ecology which, as we have seen, often involves Candida activity and increased gut permeability. The condition in the gut is summarized by one word: dysbiosis.

To help reduce intestinal dysbiosis, the following strategies are called for:

1 Probiotics (*L. acidophilus* and *Bifidobacterium*)
2 Prebiotics (FOS 4–8 g daily)
3 Foods rich in FOS (onion, asparagus, banana, Jerusalem artichoke)
4 Fibre-rich foods and/or fibre supplement (at least 40 g daily of linseed or psyllium seeds)
5 Avoidance of allergenic foods
6 Specific herbs [such as *Hydrastis canadensis* (goldenseal)]
7 Regular intake of *Allium sativum* (garlic).

Toxins which derive from a dysbiotic gut are known as endotoxins (different from toxins entering the body from outside, called exotoxins). [31] The main defence against toxicity is the liver, which undertakes hundreds of different chemical processes to achieve a toxin-free bloodstream.

The liver as the main organ of detoxification:

- filters blood
- secretes fat-soluble toxins via the bile (if there is adequate fibre)
- contains specialized cells (Kupffer cells or macrophages) which literally engulf toxins as well as deactivate larger immune complexes
- uses enzymes to take toxins apart (disassemble) and then excretes them in a complicated, two-phase operation which, if out of balance, allows highly reactive toxins to build up.

It is estimated that approximately 25 per cent of detoxification occurs in the gut itself, much of it as a result of probiotic, friendly-bacteria activity, while the remainder takes place in the liver (with water-soluble toxins leaving via the kidneys and fat-soluble ones via the bile). [19, 29]

Milk thistle herb
One of the most potent liver-supporting substances is the herb milk thistle (*Silybum marianum*). In a trial involving more than 2600 patients with a variety of liver disorders, after eight weeks of supplementation with milk thistle, over 60 per cent reported that all symptoms had disappeared (including nausea, pruritus, abdominal distention, anorexia and fatigue). Liver function tests confirmed improvement, and liver enlargement decreased. There were minimal side-effects. [32, 33]

A dose of 120 mg of silymarin three times daily has been shown to stimulate regeneration of damaged liver cells. [34]

Other liver-protecting herbs include catechin [35], dandelion root (*Taraxacum officinale*)[36] and artichoke leaves (*Cynara scolymus*). [37]

A programme of liver support is often needed before starting the anti-Candida programme fully as the process of detoxification of dying yeast as well as the possible dysbiotic state of the bowel is likely to place enormous demands on liver function.

6. IMMUNE-SYSTEM ENHANCEMENT BY SUPPLEMENTATION
To strengthen the immune system, it is suggested that a number of essential nutrients be included in the programme. As not all of these may be needed in every case, it is only by taking expert advice that your particular needs can be properly assessed.

Vitamin C

The importance of vitamin C cannot be overemphasized. T cells, which form a major part of our defence system, contain high levels of vitamin C. It has been noted that the lower the vitamin C content of these vital cells, the less efficient their performance in defending the body against intruding organisms or materials, including yeast. [38]

Any stress, whether originating in the emotions or caused by the presence of toxic pollution, infection or other factors, places demands upon vitamin C levels in the body. This is a water-soluble vitamin and the body has no stores of it, so a constant supply is needed. Research has shown a fascinating adaptation which takes place when requirements increase because of stress or infection. Under normal conditions, if a person takes more vitamin C than is actually required, a degree of diarrhoea is likely to develop. This is a well-known fact and is one way of assessing just how much vitamin C you need. If 5 g daily is taken with no resultant diarrhoea, then it can be assumed that this amount of vitamin C is needed at that time.

If, however, diarrhoea usually develops after ingesting only 2 g daily, but circumstances alter because of infection or stress, then it is possible to increase vitamin C intake to many times 2 g daily without any bowel symptoms at all. Dr Robert Cathcart has shown that, if necessary, the intake of vitamin C can be as high as 100 g a day (but never try this without supervision), with no apparent bowel sensitivity.[39]

When the crisis passes, however, such doses would produce diarrhoea, as before. Thus, the body, in its wisdom, seems to be able to alter its function to meet particular requirements in this way. To bolster a deficient immune system such as might arise with Candida spread, the recommended amount of vitamin C to be supplemented (in the absence of any bowel reaction) is 1–3 g daily with food.

Arginine

The effect of vitamin C on the T cells depends, of course, on the T cells being there to do their work. The thymus gland, which lies below the breastbone, can become relatively inactive, and one of the main nutrients which can enhance its production of T cells is the amino acid arginine.[40]

A dose of 3 g daily for a short period (say a month) will boost thymus activity at the outset of the programme, when it is most needed. Take the arginine before retiring, on an empty stomach, with water. Long-term use of arginine at these dosages is not suggested, although there are no known side-effects with doses lower than 20 g daily. Rough, thickened skin may develop on the elbows with doses above 20 g daily, but this will disappear when the supplementation is stopped. The reason for suggesting a time limit for the use of arginine is that the thymus may come to depend upon such nutritional supplementation when it should be encouraged to return to normal activity by the total programme of Candida suppression. Therefore, take 3 g daily for only the first month of the programme.

Note: If you have a history of herpes simplex infection, do *not* supplement with arginine for it has also been found to enhance herpes activity (which is countered by another amino acid, lysine).[41]

B vitamins

A further aid to the immune system is an increased intake of certain of the B vitamins.[38] It is important to the programme that these are not derived from yeast sources as anyone with a Candida problem is likely to have become yeast-sensitive. All the B vitamins are available in synthetic forms and these, rather than yeast-derived ones, are suggested in cases involving Candida.

The recommended dosages are 20–50 mg of vitamin B6 (pyridoxine), 20–50 mcg of vitamin B12 and 20–50 mcg of folic acid daily.

In addition, vitamin B5 should also be taken to assist in the enhancement of B lymphocytes, especially if there is evidence of allergic reactions or digestive involvement. This should be taken in the form of calcium pantothcnate at a dose of 500 mg daily.

Many excellent non-yeast sources of B-complex vitamins are available from all good health stores and most pharmacies.

Minerals

The minerals zinc, selenium and magnesium are all commonly implicated in deficient immune-response conditions,[42, 43] and should ideally be added to the programme. As with the B vitamins, it is important to obtain a non-yeast source of selenium. Recommended dosages (all to be taken with food) of these minerals are:

zinc (as zinc orotate, picolinate or citrate), 50 mg daily
selenium, 50 mcg daily
magnesium, 250–500 mg daily.

Finally, a supply of some of the fat-soluble vitamins is called for in our effort to resuscitate the immune response. This calls for a moderate intake of vitamin E (make sure that you buy natural vitamin E, identified by the name D-alpha-tocopherol rather than D,L-alpha-tocopherol, which is a synthetic form) at a dose of 200–400 IU (international units) daily; vitamin A in the form of beta-carotene, in a dose of up to 100,000 IU daily; and oil of evening primrose (vitamin F) in a 500-mg capsule twice daily or an alternative such as flaxseed oil.

ANTI-CANDIDA AND IMMUNE ENHANCEMENT

An important note
One or other of the antifungal approaches discussed above should be used – whether this involves tannates, caprylic acid and/or herbs such as *Berberis, Echinacea, Aloe vera* and/or garlic.

USE OF THE SUBSTANCES DISCUSSED IS AN INDIVIDUAL MATTER AND NORMALLY REQUIRES EXPERT ADVICE.
Bear in mind that whatever else is done nutritionally (*see Chapter 6*) or supplementally to enhance immune function and health, to repair the lining of the gut and to recolonize the digestive tract with friendly bacteria, there has to be an antifungal strategy to eliminate the yeast.

If you intend to self-medicate, then, at the very least, you need to take either caprylic acid, Horopeito/Mikoplex, garlic or oregano oil as well as following the immune-enhancing and probiotic supplementation suggestions, and the anti-Candida diet (*see Chapter 6*).

Anyone with a Candida problem is urged to take professional advice before embarking on an antifungal programme, however, as there are so many individual variables, and self-treatment may produce undue anxiety and disappointing results.

Note: For quantities, see the notes earlier in this chapter or discuss this with a healthcare professional (naturopath, nutritionist or pharmacist). Items marked +++ are always indicated for Candida treatment. All other substances require individualized prescribing by a suitably qualified healthcare professional.

Recolonization:

Lactobacillus acidophilus and Bifidobacterium (at least two billion viable organisms of each daily) +++

Biotin (vitamin H) +++
FOS (at least 8 g daily) +++

Antifungal agents (at least one, or a combination of several
of these, is essential):

Garlic
Aloe vera juice
Echinacea, Hydrastis and/or berberine
Pau d'arco
Polygodial (Horopeito/Mikoplex)
Caprylic acid
Oregano oil
Olive oil
Tannates
Chamomile

To enhance immune function (as indicated by history and
condition):

Vitamin C
Vitamin E
Vitamin A (as beta-carotene)
Arginine
Calcium pantothenate (vitamin B5)
Vitamin B6 (pyridoxine)
Vitamin B12
Folic acid
Or high-potency vitamin B-complex capsule (yeast-free,
slow-release, containing not less than 50 mg each of the
major B vitamins)
Selenium
Zinc
Magnesium
Oil of evening primrose (or other forms of essential
fatty acids, including flaxseed, borage and blackcurrant

seeds, as well as fish oils, may be useful under special circumstances)

Other nutrients may also be required, including:

Chromium
Iron
Manganese
Full-spectrum amino acids

Nutrient combinations including glutamine, gamma-oryzanol and NAG for healing gut mucous membrane
Liver support substances, such as milk thistle.

SIMULTANEOUS OBJECTIVES
Several strategies are needed at the same time to deal with the problems created by Candida, as explained earlier. First, we use probiotics and biotin (as well as herbal and other products as discussed) to directly inhibit Candida and fight its spread. Other nutrients are used to build up immune function (B and T cells) so that the body can better cope with the invading microorganisms. Therefore, this part of the anti-Candida programme requires taking a large number of supplements which can be both somewhat expensive and off-putting. Let it be made clear, however, that what is at stake is your health. For this reason, there should be no hesitation in grasping this opportunity to fight off the cause of your ill health by whatever safe methods are at hand. The methods being advocated here are safe as well as effective in most cases. It can take time to control Candida once it is rampant, and six months should be seen as the minimum length of time to maintain this programme.

YEAST DIE-OFF
During periods of rapid yeast destruction as the supple-mentation and dietary programme gets underway, the

body's organs of elimination (such as the liver) will be called on to detoxify the breakdown products of this process. This can lead to your feeling particularly seedy, nauseated and off-colour – a reaction known as yeast 'die-off' or 'burn-off' (or Herxheimer's reaction) – for several days or even weeks. The use of proven strains of high-potency bifidobacteria together with the general dietary strategies discussed in this and the next chapter should minimize this reaction. In any case, do not be tempted to stop the anti-Candida programme when this process becomes evident as it does not indicate that the programme is not working – indeed, quite the contrary. This is a critical stage of the treatment which, if stopped suddenly, can lead to a rebound of Candida activity and even greater feelings of ill health. This die-off period should not last for more than a week or 10 days – by which time, if you've stuck to the guidelines, a gradual improvement should be evident. Total control of the fungus and, therefore, eradication of all symptoms, can, however, take many months.

CAUTIONS AND POSSIBLE SIDE-EFFECTS OF DIETARY CHANGES

- If you have an eating disorder such as anorexia or bulimia, do not attempt to change your diet radically without expert advice and supervision.
- Expect that yeast die-off is a likely outcome that will cause odd symptoms for a week or so.
- There may be changes in bowel habits and, while these should settle down within a few weeks, seek professional advice if there is prolonged diarrhoea or constipation (increased water intake and linseed oil should normally take care of this).
- If symptoms such as palpitations, unusual fatigue, brain 'cloudiness', unusual muscle and joint discomfort or a runny nose appear, suspect a food sensitivity and carefully analyse anything new in your diet; use

exclusion and rotation (as discussed for yeast; *see Chapter 6*) to identify any culprit foods or substances, which should then be excluded for at least three months.

- Expect that any local yeast-affected areas will become worse for a few days. This includes oral, vaginal and skin areas. This will calm down on its own, but can be helped by the use of local treatment methods (discussed below).

- Do not be surprised if you start to crave foods (sugars and starches in particular). This is usually a result of an imbalance in blood-sugar levels due to the dietary changes and should settle down in time. If the craving is bothersome or severe, either take expert advice or use one of the following tactics to help balance blood-sugar levels:

  - Take 1 g daily of the amino-acid L-glutamine (away from mealtimes) and assess its effect on the craving
  - Supplement with 3–4 g of full-spectrum amino acids (Lamberts' Protein Build is recommended) between meals, two or three times daily
  - Take one Glucose Tolerance Factor tablet daily (containing 200 mcg of chromium)
  - Eat little and often (from the list of appropriate foods in Chapter 6), with snacks between meals and one late at night before bedtime.

LOCAL VAGINAL ANTI-CANDIDA TREATMENT

A number of approaches may be useful for soothing inflamed vaginal tissues during anti-Candida treatment. Whichever is used, it is imperative that a comprehensive antifungal dietary approach is also followed, or a recurrence of thrush or yeast-caused vaginitis will be very likely.

1 Using a special soft-tipped disposable applicator, insert a solution of high-potency *L. acidophilus* culture

mixed with pure water or, even better, some diluted *Aloe vera* juice. Any of the acidophilus products recommended for dietary use can be used in this way. Another way to achieve this effect is to puncture an acidophilus capsule with several pin-pricks and to insert the capsule deep into the vagina overnight. The acidophilus will leak out of the capsule and inhibit the yeast, and the empty capsule can be expelled by douching (*see below*). Alternatively, you can mix a teaspoonful of acidophilus powder or the contents of two capsules with live yoghurt and insert this into the vagina overnight, although this will be messy. Finally, douching with water containing a teaspoonful of dissolved acidophilus powder will also be effective.

2 Aloe vera juice alone (two teaspoonfuls diluted in a half-pint of water) can be used as a douche to relieve itching and burning.

3 A cream derived from mountain ash berries (*Sorbus aucuparia*) has been shown to have powerful antifungal and soothing properties when applied locally into or onto the vagina (marketed in the UK as Cervagyn). The active constituent, potassium sorbate, is a common food preservative (antifungal agent) which, in much higher concentrations, can prevent yeast proliferation by interfering with its ability to feed off carbohydrates (sugars). In a study of 37 women with vulvovaginitis using potassium sorbate in a 1 per cent strength, there were only 11 recurrences of candidiasis over a three-month period. When a 3 per cent solution was used, there were no recurrences in any of the 32 women participating in the study after six months. There was also rapid symptomatic relief when yeast was the sole infecting agent. Where other microorganisms were involved, other methods were

needed. The results were uniformly better when the diets of the women involved were low in sugar of any kind.

4 Tannate extracts are also available (from healthfood stores) for use as a douche. This combines irreversibly with yeast cells, deactivating them and also preventing their adherence to the walls of the vagina.

5 Tea tree oil used as a pessary or diluted in water as a douche is an effective (if slightly irritating at first) antifungal treatment for any vaginitis of yeast origin.

6 Dilute vinegar (or lemon juice) douches, on their own or with acidophilus powder added, are useful for soothing irritated vaginal tissues and for acidifying the area. A more acidic environment is supportive of friendly bacteria and makes it more difficult for yeast to adhere to the vaginal walls. *Never* use vinegar neat on these sensitive tissues.

7 Soothing antifungal *Calendula* (marigold) pessaries are available at some specialist healthfood outlets.

COLONIC IRRIGATION AND ENEMAS
Colonic irrigation involves the administration of water into the bowel that is sometimes combined with other substances to clear debris from the region and to encourage its health. Useful in this respect are added garlic extract, oxygen and acidophilus. Periodic applications of water coupled with one of these additives can greatly improve the condition of the bowel. Enemas are less effective since they penetrate only a short distance, unlike the colonic, which can pass water along the entire length of the large bowel. The technique requires expert skills, and its use for Candida problems requires additional knowledge. In principle, however, such treatment is recommended at least in the early stages of the programme.

However, a caution is required regarding excessive use of colonic irrigation since it can actually deplete the normal flora if done too frequently. Its use should be limited to an actual need, a precise prescription of the number of applications and, essentially, for reimplantation of friendly organisms as part of the process.

YEAST DESENSITIZATION AS A WAY TO CONTROL CANDIDA

Carefully controlled doses of Candida extract may be injected in an attempt to produce an immune-system response. Antibodies thus produced by white blood cells can assist in the defence against antigens entering the system because of the yeast. The use of yeast extracts as a 'vaccine' of sorts also appears to assist general immune function by helping to balance or regulate aspects the production of 'helper' and 'suppressor' cells, as discussed earlier (*see Chapter 2*).

However, this whole procedure is extremely complicated because, although *Candida albicans* is a clearly identifiable strain of yeast, it contains a large number of variables. Thus, the Candida which is growing in one person is never exactly the same as that growing in another. This biological individuality applies to yeasts as much as it does to every other living creature, including people (*see the discussion of blood types in Chapters 2 and 3*). Therefore, injecting the same extract of Candida into two different people will not produce the same response, nor is the yeast likely to be the same as that to which the individual is normally exposed, so this is a process of trial and error. Genetic factors may be largely responsible for the different responses of individuals to such treatment, so anti-Candida desensitization treatment needs to be applied by an expert in the field who is able to cope with all the complex variables.

Even should such expertise be available, this approach, with all its possible pitfalls in terms of variable reactions, at best can only deal with just one aspect of the problem. It may assist in bolstering the immune system against the byproducts of Candida infestation, which is especially desirable for those who are suffering from the type of allergy symptoms mentioned earlier, but it will do little for the local symptoms currently active in the bowel or reproductive system. Only those harmful effects of Candida that are mediated by the bloodstream will be helped by this procedure. Valuable as that may be, it would leave much of the underlying condition untouched, and would still require a programme of anti-Candida diet and supplements to control its spread and feeding.

Truss points out that the use of this type of 'vaccination' programme is contraindicated in patients suffering from what are called autoimmune conditions, including rheumatoid arthritis. Stimulation of the immune response in someone who is being attacked by his or her own immune system would lead to aggravation of the condition. As Truss has written: 'I obtain yeast from supply houses that have been made aware of the necessity of bioassaying each new batch on humans. Prior to their being informed of this fact, they were putting out a number of batches that would not give a positive skin test on known reactors. The preparation as I order it is simply *Candida albicans* 1:10.'[44]

This indicates one more pitfall in this method: it is vital that the Candida extract used is actually active and this needs to be proven with each batch produced, otherwise the pitfalls described above are compounded.

Before moving to the next chapter, here is a summary of the main medical antifungal treatments. This is provided for information rather than as a recommendation for the use of these products, many of which are known to produce undesirable side-effects.

MEDICAL ANTIFUNGAL STRATEGIES

The orthodox medical drug treatment of fungal infection, such as Candida, involves the use of antifungal antibiotics such as nystatin. This drug is active against a wide range of yeasts and yeast-like fungi, including Candida, and comes in a variety of forms – as a liquid for use in the mouth, as tablets for use in treating Candida in the intestinal tract, as suppositories for use in the vagina, and as creams, ointments and powders for the treatment of surface areas such as the skin and nails.

Some of the reasons for urging caution with the long-term use of nystatin have been given in earlier chapters. Nystatin is suggested as a safe and helpful drug by authorities such as Dr William Crook, whose book *The Yeast Connection* has done so much to encourage awareness of the damage candidiasis can cause. Nystatin is lethal to yeast cells on contact. Getting them into contact with the drug is not always easy, especially if they are deep in the bowel. Also, nystatin passing through the bowel will kill all surface yeasts, but none that are embedded deeper into the walls of the intestine. In fact, despite assurances from Crook and other experts that nystatin only acts within the digestive tract, it seems likely that, where the gut wall has been damaged by yeast (increased permeability or leaky gut syndrome), some of the drug may enter the bloodstream with unpredictable results.

Activist author Gill Jacobs points out another possibility in her excellent book *Candida albicans: A User's Guide to Treatment and Recovery* – that nystatin is a polyene antibiotic and such substances have been found to actually boost the numbers of yeast cells that can colonize our tissues.[45]

OTHER ANTIFUNGAL DRUGS

There are a number of other commonly used antifungal drugs which have various drawbacks compared with the safer, natural substances discussed in this book.

Diflucan (fluconazole)
This expensive drug requires lengthy use to have any noticeable effects.

Amphotericin B
Known as fungalin, this has similarities with nystatin. Banned in the USA, it is known to be toxic when used intravenously, which must raise doubts regarding safety because of the possibility of absorption through a damaged gut wall.

Nizoral (ketoconazole)
Nizoral causes damage to the liver as a result of its easy access to the bloodstream from the intestinal tract.

In medical settings, none of these drugs is generally used with a comprehensive antifungal dietary and supplement approach to encourage a healthier digestive tract and immune system. None of these drugs are usually necessary since the methods outlined in this book are safer and of proven efficacy. If a condition such as Candida has become so widespread as to cause a problem, then it is vital that the immune system and bowel flora, which should be controlling the situation, are revitalized. Reliance on nystatin or any other drug will leave the immune system in the same depleted state except that there will be, over a period of time, fewer yeast byproducts entering the bloodstream to challenge the immune system. This, it is thought (by experts such as Drs Truss and Crook), allows the immune system to revive gradually.

There is certainly no objection to nystatin being employed if the condition is severe enough to warrant it, but this should only be done in combination with the sort of programme outlined in this book. Otherwise, there will be only short-term gains and the condition will recur. It is important to realize that nystatin is itself derived from a mould and can cause allergic symptoms in some yeast-sensitive individuals. Some patients become dependent on nystatin and find it difficult to be weaned off it. One of the more distressing factors relating to long-term use of nystatin is the likelihood of a 'rebound' of yeast activity when it is stopped.

By relying on a supplementation programme as outlined here, together with the dietary guidelines in Chapter 6, it is possible to not only control Candida, but to improve your general wellbeing dramatically. This is something no drug can achieve, whether it produces side-effects or not.

Our next consideration is the importance of combining the supplemental attack on Candida, healing of the gut wall, detoxification and enhancement of the immune system with a dietary programme that deprives the yeast of its main source of food – sugar.

REFERENCES

1 Crook W. *The Yeast Connection*, Jackson, TN: Professional Books, 1988
2 Pizzorno J, Murray M, Joiner-Bey H. *Clinician's Handbook of Natural Medicine*, London: Churchill Livingstone, 2002
3 Miles M *et al.* 'Recurrent candidiasis: importance of intestinal reservoir', *JAMA* 1977; 238: 1836–7
4 Nystatin Multicenter Study Group. 'Therapy of candidal vaginitis: the effect of eliminating intestinal Candida', *Am J Obstet Gynecol* 1986; 155: 651–4
5 Winderlin C, Sehnert K. *Candida-Related Complex: What Your Doctor Might Be Missing*, Taylor Publishing, 1996
6 Spinillo A *et al.* 'Effect of antibiotic use on the prevalence of symptomatic vulvovaginal candidiasis', *Am J Obstet Gynecol* 1999; 180: 14–17
7 Neuhauser I. 'Successful treatment of intestinal moniliasis with fatty acid resin complex', *Arch Intern Med* 1954; 93: 53–60

8 Marz RB. *Medical Nutrition From Marz*, 2nd edn, Portland, OR: Omni Press, 1997

9 Tadi P. 'Anticandidal and anticarcinogenic potentials for garlic', *Int Clin Nutr Rev* 1990; 10(4): 423–9

10 *Med J Aust* 1982; 1: 60

11 *Mycologia* 1975; LXVII (4)

12 *Mycologia* 1977; LXIX (4)

13 Mahajan V *et al.* 'Antimycotic activity of berberine sulphate', *Sabouraudia* 1982; 20: 79–81

14 Amin AH *et al.* 'Berberine sulfate: antimicrobial activity, bioassay, and mode of action', *Can J Microbiol* 1969; 15: 1067–76

15 For research documentation, see enquiries@forestherbs.co.nz

16 Stiles J. 'The inhibition of Candida albicans by oregano', *J Appl Nutr* 1995; 47: 96–102

17 Hammer KA *et al.* 'Antimicrobial activity of essential oils and other plant extracts', *J Appl Microbiol* 1999; 86: 985–90

18 Talpur N *et al.* 'Medicinal herbal oils: antifungal effects of the edible oil of oregano', *J Am Coll Nutr*, 2000; 19 (5): 689

19 Pizzorno J, Murray M. 'Tabebuia avellanedae', *Textbook of Natural Medicine*, Edinburgh: Churchill Livingstone, 2001

20 Bland J. *J Alt Med*, 1985: June

21 Yamaguchi H. 'Mycelial development and chemical alteration of *Candida albicans* from biotin insufficiency', *Sabouraudia* 1974; 12: 320–8

22 Gibson GR, Berry Ottaway P, Rastall RA. *Prebiotics: New Developments in Functional Foods*, Oxford: Chandos Publishing, 2000

23 Gibson GR, Roberfroid MB. 'Dietary modulation of the human colonic microbiota: introducing the concept of prebiotics', *J Nutr* 1995; 125: 1401–12

24 Shehani K. 'Role of dietary lactobacilli in gastrointestinal microecology', *Am J Clin Nutr* 1980; 33: 2448–57

25 Kageyama T *et al.* 'The effect of bifidobacterium administration in patients with leukemia', *Bifidobacteria Microflora* 1984; 3: 29–33

26 Bland J. '*Candida albicans*: an alternative therapy for an unexpected problem', *J Alt Med* 1983; July: 8–19

27 Gilliland S *et al.* 'Beneficial interrelationships between certain micro-organisms and humans', *J Food Protect* 1979; 42: 164–7

28 Stock S. 'Conquering Candida', *J Alt Complement Med*, 1993; June: 25

29 Martinez-Gonzalez O *et al.* 'Intestinal permeability in patients with ankylosing spondylitis', *Br J Rheumatol* 1994; 33: 644–7

30 Paganelli R *et al.* 'Intestinal permeability in patients with urticaria-angiodema', *Ann Allergy* 1991; 66: 181–4

31 Pizzorno J. *Total Wellness*, Rocklin CA: Prima Publishing, 1996

32 Salmi H. 'Effects of silymarin on chemical, functional and morphological alterations of the liver: A double-blind controlled study', *Scand J Gastroenterol* 1982; 17: 417–21

33 Albrecht M *et al.* 'Therapy of toxic liver pathologies with Legalon', *Z Klin Med* 1992; 47: 87–92

34 Wagner H. 'Antihepatotoxic flavonoids', Cody V et al. (eds), *Plant Flavonoids in Biology and Medicine*, New York: Alan R. Liss, 1986

35 World M *et al.* 'Cyanidanol-3 for alcoholic liver disease: six months' clinical trial', *Alcohol Alcoholism* 1984; 19: 23–9

36 Faber K. 'The dandelion: Taraxacum officinale', *Weber Pharm* 1991; 13: 423–35

37 Kirchoff R *et al.* 'Increase in choleresis by means of artichoke extract', *Phytomedicine* 1994; 1: 107–15

38 Bland J. *Nutraerobics*, New York: Harper & Row, 1983

39 Cathcart R. 'Vitamin C: titrating to bowel tolerance',
    Med Hypoth 1981; 7: 1359–76

40 *Am J Clin Nutr* 1983; 37 (5): 786

41 *Dermatologia* 1978; 156: 257–67

42 Bland J (ed). *Medical Application of Clinical
    Nutrition*, New Canaan, CN: Keats Publishing, 1983

43 Edman J *et al.* 'Zinc status in women with
    vulvovaginal candidiasis', *Am J Obstet Gynecol* 1986;
    155: 1082–6

44 Truss C. *The Missing Diagnosis*, Birmingham, AL:
    Self-published, 1980

45 Jacobs G. *Candida albicans: A User's Guide to
    Treatment and Recovery*, London: Optima, 1994: 23

6 | *The anti-Candida diet*

Before examining dietary strategies related to Candida problems, it is important to comment on the need for a sound environment for digestion in the stomach. Many people who suffer from 'dyspepsia' and 'heartburn' are not, in fact, the victims of excessive acid, but of too little, and their symptoms represent what happens when:

1   food is not adequately digested in the stomach, leading to excessive fermentation and gas, and

2   there is activity of yeast in an environment which is not sufficiently acidic to inhibit them.

In 1985, researchers showed that *Candida albicans* needs a slightly alkaline environment to thrive (pH of 7.4) and, in a strongly acid environment (pH of 4.5), it is completely inactivated. People taking antacid medication may therefore be encouraging yeast activity in their stomach and digestive tract.[1]

Dr Stephen Davies, in his book *Nutritional Medicine* (Pan, 1989), lists some of the common conditions associated with too little hydrochloric (stomach) acid, including asthma, food allergy, iron and vitamin B12 deficiency (and therefore fatigue), bacterial and yeast bowel overgrowth, arthritic symptoms, diabetes, underactive thyroid gland, bowel sensitivity and eczema.

Among the causes of inadequate acid secretion in the stomach can be exposure to toxic pollution (such as DDT), marijuana smoking and excessive coffee consumption – and deficiency of the mineral zinc, essential for the body to make adequate stomach acids.

As a first step in normalizing such a problem, a strategy can be used in which hydrochloric acid capsules (betaine hydrochloride) are taken with each meal.[2] If this eases symptoms significantly, then a herbal method for stimulating the production of digestive acid is suggested, which involves taking of a teaspoonful of Swedish bitters (a combination of herbs such as dandelion) two or three times daily, about 20 minutes before eating. A test which measures the levels of zinc in sweat can show clearly whether there is a deficiency and, thus, whether supplementation is needed. If you are zinc-deficient, a dose of approximately 20 mg daily taken for several months should replenish this vital mineral.

Digestive enzymes

A second digestive strategy may also prove useful especially if food intolerance or allergy is a feature of your condition. This calls for supplementation with natural enzymes – chemicals which assist in the breakdown of food. Enzymes may be inadequately available for a variety of reasons. A broad-spectrum enzyme combination is suggested for anyone with sensitivity or allergy symptoms.[3]

If bloating and 'acid-stomach' symptoms are also a feature of an allergic condition, then supplementation with betaine hydrochloride and/or Swedish bitters (*see above*).

Two main strategies

There are two primary dietary approaches which have to be considered in treating Candida overgrowth. The first and most important involves sugar exclusion from the diet (*see pages 118–22*). This approach applies to everyone with a Candida problem, without exception, and is among the most important elements in controlling its activity. The second strategy is appropriate if there is the possibility that you may have become sensitized (or 'allergic') to yeast and its byproducts because of your Candida problem.[4] As already explained, this is more likely if your condition is chronic and ongoing, and if the mucous membrane of your intestinal tract has been irritated or even damaged by the invasive fungal form of Candida.

If this is the case, then avoidance of foods derived from yeast or contaminated with mould is essential for a period of months. The guidelines for achieving a yeast-free diet are explained below.

A strategy used by some practitioners, called 'desensitization', uses minute dilutions of yeasts to reduce this sort of allergic reaction (and is described at the end of Chapter 5 for information only as it is a complicated, expensive and not always successful procedure). It is important, however, that you arc awarc of this option as it has helped many people who have become 'super-allergic', and some allergy experts might recommend the method.

Both Drs Truss and Crook strongly advocate the dietary approach to treatment of Candida, especially for the prevention of Candida spread. They are also supportive of desensitization methods.

My own view is that the dietary approach (*see page 114*) combined with the anti-Candida methods described in Chapter 5 offer the best and safest way forward for anyone with a health problem caused by aggressive yeast overgrowth.

Foods derived from or containing fungi and yeast

The following is a list of foods and substances containing yeast or yeast-like substances, and so should be avoided as much as possible during the initial stages of dealing with Candida infection by anyone who is sensitive to them. It is probably wise to maintain vigilance concerning these foods for at least three months; after that time, a degree of relaxation can be exercised – with the proviso that, if such foods are reintroduced and symptoms which had been quiescent become active again, you will once again eliminate yeast-related foods and return to a stricter mode of eating for a while.

The rationale behind such avoidance is that, in practice, these foods appear to aggravate a Candida-induced condition, especially if allergic symptoms are part of the picture, and there are symptoms such as bloating and intestinal gas.[5]

In a letter to me, Dr Truss states:

'If someone has no symptoms, I see no reason to have him avoid these yeast-promoting foods, although I will say that in excess, and combined with a high-carbohydrate intake [sugars, etc.], these may actually induce this condition [Candida infection] even without the stimulatory effects of antibiotics, birth-control pills, cortisone, etc.'

Is there any proof of the value of such restrictions? Space does not permit discussion of all the information proving that these restrictions are valid ways of reducing the load on the immune system brought about by repetitive allergic or sensitivity reactions, but the details of one report show their potential.

In a study of 50 patients with chronic urticaria (an allergic skin condition), all of whom had Candida antigens in their blood, it was found that more than half reacted (with acute skin eruptions) to yeast supplements, and over half were said to be 'clinically cured' of their condition after following a low-yeast diet and antifungal therapy.[6]

When individuals are yeast-sensitive/-allergic, it is often found that they have a reaction to a wide range of fungi from many possible sources.[7] It is best, therefore, to eliminate these in the early stages of the programme to reduce stress on immune function.

Yeast-containing foods and substances

The following foods contain yeast as an added ingredient in their preparations[8] and may therefore be undesirable, especially in the early stages of an anti-Candida programme:

> yeast spreads (such as Marmite)
> breads (non-yeasted wholewheat, soda bread or corn bread is usually acceptable unless there is a grain sensitivity)
> cakes and cake mixes
> biscuits and crackers
> enriched flour
> buns, rolls and pastries
> anything fried in breadcrumbs (such as fish fingers).

The following contain yeast or yeast-like substances because of their inherent nature or the way in which they are manufactured:

> mushrooms
> truffles
> soy sauce
> stock and soup cubes

buttermilk and sour cream
black tea
all cheeses (especially aged or blue cheeses), including
cottage cheese (although some experts allow this)
citrus drinks if canned or frozen
all dried fruits (high mould presence on their surfaces)
all fermented beverages, such as beer, spirits, wine,
cider and ginger ale
all malted products (cereals, sweets or dairy products
which have been malted)
all foods containing monosodium glutamate (which is
often a yeast derivative)
all vinegars, whether grape, malt, cider or anything else
(frequently used in sauces and relishes as well as in
salad dressings, sauerkraut, olives and pickled foods).

NOTE: There is disagreement among experts as to the wisdom of excluding vinegar and similar products (sauerkraut,
pickles, olives) from an anti-Candida diet, and there are certainly benefits to be gained by taking apple-cider vinegar –
but only if no negative reactions are observed. A simple test
would be to introduce this in a teaspoon in warm water two
or three times daily and keep a careful note of any changes
in your symptoms (*see Chapter 7 for details of how to keep
a symptom score sheet*).

The following are either derived from yeast or contain
elements derived from it, and so should be avoided for at
least the first three months of the anti-Candida regime if
you show any sign of a sensitivity to yeasts or moulds:

some antibiotics
multivitamin tablets (unless they specifically state they
are from a non-yeast source)
B-complex vitamins (*see Chapter 5*)
selenium (*see Chapter 5*)
individual B vitamins (*see Chapter 5*).

Dr Truss singles out some foods from this long list as the main culprits. He states:

'It is my belief that there are several foods that are primarily to be avoided. These include all fermented drinks as well as vinegar, mushrooms and mouldy cheeses. I allow my patients to have cottage cheese as well as yoghurt.'

Furthermore, he says:

'It is rational to remove all of these foods from the diet only if there is an indication that patients are having trouble with [the] yeast, Candida.'[9]

Elimination/challenge/rotation

If you have any doubts as to whether any of these foods are likely to be a problem for you, then there are two different ways to test this.

1 You should eliminate that food for at least one week, then reintroduce it twice in one day. If no reaction occurs, such as immediate palpitations, sudden fatigue or unusual brain 'cloudiness', or no return over the next 24 hours of symptoms which have been absent or quiescent, then you can probably include that food into your diet once more. The safest way to do this would be in a rotation pattern where you eat the food no more than once every four or five days until the programme is well established, say after three months.

2 You should eliminate the food (or the entire food 'family' such as dairy, grains or yeasts) for a week, then reintroduce the foods into your normal diet for

several weeks. Once again, you should monitor your symptoms (*see Chapter 7 for details of how to record symptom scores*). If you felt better (had reduced symptom scores) after a week of avoidance of the food(s) and started to develop the symptoms again after a few days of eating it/them again, this is confirmation that the food(s) should be eliminated for several months before attempting them again.

If you are truly sensitized to a particular food, you may have withdrawal symptoms during the first few days of avoidance. This is normal and tells you in advance that the foods you have left out of your diet have been harming you and distressing your immune system. The (almost complete) elimination of all yeast-based foods, alcoholic beverages and vinegar (and its byproducts as listed) as well as giving up blue cheeses and mushrooms comprise one part of the major dietary changes required for the first few months. The other key changes involve the elimination/reduction of intake of refined carbohydrates and foods rich in sugar.

Sugar-rich foods

Sugar (sucrose) itself, in whatever guise, is to be strictly avoided during the battle to control Candida. This means white sugar, brown sugar, black sugar and all shades in between. There is no such thing as a healthy sugar. We do not need sugar as such for health. Its sole claim for desirability is its taste, which it is relatively easy to learn to do without. All sugars will aid the growth and proliferation of yeast. This includes syrups, honey (yes, I'm afraid so) and other forms of sugar such as fructose, maltose, glucose or sorbitol, molasses, date sugar, maple sugar and the whole range of non-foods with which our real foods and beverages have been sweetened. Sweets, chocolates and all soft drinks should also be avoided.

The inclusion of honey may come as a surprise. I myself had assumed that honey was relatively safe as, to my knowledge, it did not become mouldy. In this I was corrected by Dr Truss, who communicated the fact that honey does indeed contain yeast spores: 'Species of *Zygosaccharomyces*, a yeast, have been found particularly active in causing yeast spoilage of honey.'

It is known that honey is hygroscopic (it absorbs water) and that, at a certain degree of moisture content, there will be sufficient water at the surface to dilute the concentration of sugars to a point where the yeasts and bacteria which might be present can grow. Thus, yeasts and other microorganisms capable of surviving in concentrated sugar solutions (in which no yeast will grow) become able to thrive, given a certain degree of dilution. To prevent this from happening, honey is heated and often has additives such as sodium benzoate mixed with it to inhibit the growth of fermenting yeasts.

Truss and Crook both insist that honey be included in the list of banned foods during an anti-Candida campaign. The length of time that this will be necessary depends on the speed of your recovery – probably not less than three months and more likely to be six.

The undesirability of eating yeast-containing foods removes bread, pastry, biscuits and cakes. This is doubly necessary since these foods have a high content of refined carbohydrates (unless totally wholegrain). Any carbohydrate that has been refined beyond the simple grinding stage is undesirable. Wholewheat, porridge oats, millet or brown rice are all highly desirable foods that are rich in what are known as complex carbohydrates. These should (especially oats) be a part of the diet. Once these are broken down into fine flours and are refined further, they become less desirable, becoming food for the yeast rather than for you.

So, even in the middle stages of the programme when, hopefully, your symptoms are easing and you may justifiably feel that you can relax the stricter aspects of the diet, please remember that refined carbohydrates are the natural food of yeast, and Candida will thank you for delivering such foods by a rapid expansion of its activity.

As Truss puts it:

'Decreased availability of carbohydrates slows the rate of multiplication of yeast cells, and thus should reduce the amount of yeast products entering the bloodstream.'

The opposite is also true: the more of these foods there are in the diet, the greater will the chances be of further spread of Candida. So, out of the diet goes everything – flour products of all sorts, biscuits, cakes, buns, rolls and bread (unless made with wholegrains and without yeast or sugar, such as soda bread) – but wholemeal pasta and pastry.

Many foods have 'hidden sugar' in that sugar is added during the processing or preparation. These are often foods with which sugar is not usually associated – such as frozen peas, most canned foods, and many packaged and processed foods. These all contain either refined flour products or sugar, or both. For this reason, and for the general undesirability of many such foods from a nutritional viewpoint, these should be avoided. Otherwise, not only are you providing the favourite foods of the yeasts within your body when you eat sugar, you are also causing a degree of metabolic and physiological mayhem.

It should be recalled that, until about a hundred years ago, the average annual intake of sugar in Western countries was around 9 kg (20 lb) per head, and this was part of a dietary pattern which included far more 'natural' vitamin- and mineral-rich foods than is currently the case. The present annual intake of sugar in the UK and USA is over 45 kg (100 lb) per head of the population. The human body is very adaptable, but it takes more than a century to get used to such a change in nutritional intake.

Organs such as the pancreas (the source of insulin and essential protein-digesting enzymes) are grossly over-worked when sugar plays a large part in the diet. The pancreas, when faced with sugar, pumps out insulin, which has the job of maintaining the proper level of sugar in the bloodstream. Insulin is also released in response to stimulant drinks, such as coffee and tea, which initially cause the liver to release its stored sugar (as does stress). Thus, a diet rich in sugar and containing the usual tea, coffee and alcohol (as well as cola drinks and chocolates, which also contain caffeine to stimulate this cycle) will produce a situation in which a major organ is grossly overworked. In this pattern, the fluctuations in blood-sugar levels – boosted by dietary sugar and the sugar released from the liver, then depressed and controlled by the pancreatic insulin – have a profound effect upon a person's health and personality. Stress also produces the release of adrenaline and, therefore, increases sugar in the bloodstream, hence the need for as calm a state as possible to enhance health.

A sugar-rich diet also makes it much less likely that an individual will eat foods rich in vitamins and minerals sufficient to meet the minimum standards of nutrition. Thus, other systems in the body become deficient, including the immune system. This whole process may take years, all the while accompanied by a declining sense of wellbeing and an unseen rise in Candida activity. Sugar is well described as 'pure, white and deadly'.

It is suggested that, in the first few weeks of the anti-Candida programme (say, three weeks to be safe), even fresh fruit should be avoided because of its high content of natural fruit sugars. And even when fruit is resumed after the three-week break, it should exclude very sweet melons, apples and grapes, which are too high in sugar for the Candida sufferer (and often contain surface moulds).

Milk contains its own form of sugar and this, too, is thought to be undesirable throughout the programme. Pasteurized milk encourages Candida.[10] The exception to this is yoghurt if it is 'natural and live', which should be clearly stated on the container. There are many 'dead' yoghurts about and a good many have added sugar – these are unsuitable to the programme. Yoghurt itself is helpful since (if 'live') it contains bacteria which inhibit Candida and assist in the repopulation of the 'friendly' gut flora.

Does a low-sugar diet help control yeast infection?

In one study of 100 women with Candida-induced vaginitis, it was found that the levels of glucose and other sugar breakdown products excreted correlated well with the amount of dairy products, artificial sweeteners and sugars the women consumed. When they were placed on a diet which eliminated these, there were 'dramatic reductions in the incidence and severity of their illness'.[11, 12]

In another study, it was shown that *Candida albicans* could not grow in human saliva until sugar (glucose) was added.[13]

Other foods to avoid

It is best to avoid smoked meats and fish, sausages, corned beef, hot dogs and hamburgers because they all contain added substances, some of which derive from yeasts. Nuts, other than freshly cracked ones, should also be avoided because of the mould that these attract as they become rancid. Any foods which have been kept for a while other than in a frozen state are liable to be slightly mouldy, and these should be avoided too.

You now have a picture of the type of foods not to eat: mainly, the yeast- and fungus-related foods as well as refined carbohydrates and anything containing them.

Motivation

The degree to which such a programme is adhered to depends on many factors, but none less than motivation. Just how much do you want to get better, and how much effort are you prepared to put into that quest? It is completely up to you.

Certainly, taking supplements as described here will go a long way towards that end, as will avoiding yeasts and the foods derived from them. But putting the whole programme together, including the sugar-free part of the diet, will give the whole process a chance to work quickly and well.

What you can still eat is varied and exciting. Below is a pattern of eating which is nutritious, tasty and, above all, 'anti-Candida'. Once you have followed this pattern of eating for a while, it is unlikely you will ever want to reintroduce most of the 'undesirables', even when Candida is back under control.

Recommended dietary pattern

BREAKFAST
It has been found that a high-fibre diet is best suited to the resolution of the Candida problem. In the words of Professor Jeffrey Bland:

'The diet should be higher than normal in fibre, using oat bran fibre to increase the absorptive surface of the faecal material and also hasten the elimination of metabolic by-products.'[14]

It is also suggested that you eat three meals a day, and do not skip a meal unless you are feeling off-colour and have no appetite. Choose from the following for a wholesome and non-Candida-supporting breakfast:

1 Oatmeal porridge. Add a little cinnamon and some freshly ground cashew nuts for additional flavour. Use no sugar or honey. Make with water, not milk. You can add several spoonfuls of FOS, which has a slightly sweet taste, to feed your friendly bacteria (*see Chapter 5*).

2 Mixed seed and nut breakfast (combine sunflowerseeds, pumpkinseeds, sesame seeds and linseed together with oatmeal or flaked millet). This can be eaten as they are or soaked overnight in a little water to give it a softer texture, or moistened with natural live yoghurt. Add wheatgerm and freshly milled nuts, and FOS, if desired.

3 On alternate days: two eggs, any style except raw.

4 Bread or toast (made without yeast or sugar) with butter or olive oil.

5 Brown rice kedgeree (with fish).

6 Wholewheat or rice and oat pancakes (no sweetening; add FOS if you wish).

7 Natural live yoghurt (low-fat if possible) or 'virtually fat-free' fromage frais, to which is added a dessert-spoonful of cold-pressed flaxseed oil; blend well, then

add linseed and other seeds, and some FOS. This makes an energy-rich 'power breakfast' and is highly recommended (as long as you have no sensitivity to dairy products).

8 After the first three weeks or so of the programme, fresh fruit can be added to the menu – for example, sliced banana, grated apple or other fresh fruit may be added to items 1, 2 or 7, or fruit may be eaten as a major part of the meal with a handful of nuts (fresh) and/or seeds (such as sunflowerseeds or pumpkin-seeds). However, continue to avoid fruit juices.

9 Fish (not smoked) or meat (not cured or salted).

10 Wholewheat or whole-rice flakes and yoghurt (ensure there is no sugar in cereals). Use muesli-type breakfast mixtures only if they are home-made. If ready-made, they will contain dried fruit and nuts of almost certain rancidity, and frequently with added sugar or honey as well. By simply mixing oat or millet flakes with fresh nuts or seeds (*see item* 2), it is possible to make your own high-fibre, nutritious and tasty mix. Items 1 and 2 both ensure a high-fibre content, and these are suggested as the most desirable. With any of the other choices, add a heaped teaspoonful of linseed and bran (50:50 ratio) to the meal, or swallow it separately at the end of the meal with a little water.

CHEW!

Remember to chew all food thoroughly, especially carbohydrates. Half-chewed carbohydrates cannot be digested since the enzymes present in saliva are essential for the breakdown of these foods. For this reason, it is also undesirable to drink during a meal as the liquid is frequently used to facilitate swallowing, thereby reducing the need for efficient chewing. A high-fibre meal is ideal for an anti-Candida programme. It also ensures a steady release of natural sugars into the bloodstream rather than the rapid rise produced by most refined sugar-rich foods. This helps to keep blood-sugar levels even, and avoids the ups and downs in available energy (and mood) that may be a major cause of the craving for a 'quick sugar-fix'.

Drinks at breakfast time should be either green tea, pau d'arco tea, China tea or herb tea (such as Rooibosch or chamomile) – all unsweetened – or mineral water, not fruit juices unless diluted 50:50 with water and, even then, not for the first two to three weeks of the programme.

It is also suggested that, in addition to other liquids, you drink not less than 1.5 litres – and ideally up to 2.5 litres – of spring or filtered water daily, mainly away from meal-times.

MAIN MEALS

There is no reason not to be able to eat splendid food even during the strict avoidance period of the dietary programme, although one area of contention is the choice of animal proteins. The subject of blood type and whether, for genetic reasons, some people 'should' eat meat or not remains controversial. In my opinion, blood type and secretor status should be considered. Some people are natural mixed feeders, others natural vegetarians and still others may benefit from a high intake of animal protein. For more information on the concepts of individual susceptibility relating to blood types and secretor status, see Peter D'Adamo's book *Live Right for Your Type*.

ANIMAL PROTEIN

It is important to remember that most commercial meat, poultry and eggs contain residues of antibiotics and hormonal substances which were fed to the animals while rearing them for market. This means that eating beef, pork or chicken on a regular basis is a potential danger to the success of the whole programme (and a health hazard at all times), unless it comes from a source known to avoid such methods. Indeed, it is not improbable that this is a major, but as yet unrecognized, factor in the whole Candida scenario. While the use of antibiotics and steroids in medication can be relatively easily remembered and identified in the medical history, it is impossible to know just how much of these same substances are being ingested on a daily basis through food.

Thus, it is suggested that efforts be made to track down non-steroid-fed meat, poultry and eggs (and non-farmed fish) in which antibiotics have not been used. In major cities, this is probably possible. Some shops will guarantee supplies of meats and poultry free of all contamination. Lamb and mutton are less likely to be affected by this sort of additive, as are rabbit and other game meat or poultry. Fish is usually safe, apart from other sources of pollution which do not concern Candida directly and farmed fish, which may also have antibiotic contamination. For the duration of the diet, it is suggested that unless the source of fish, meat or poultry can be certainly identified as free of hormones or antibiotics, meat should be limited to game, rabbit (unless 'farmed'), mutton, lamb and fish from 'wild' sources.

VEGETABLES

Ideally, to maintain the high-fibre type of meal that is so desirable when Candida is active, the two main meals of the day should include as wide a variety of fresh vegetables as possible. Remember to eat as much of the oligosaccharide (FOS)-containing vegetables as possible (*see Chapter 5*), including onion, leek, asparagus, garlic and Jerusalem artichoke (as well as bananas, which are also rich in FOS).

It is often the case that a digestive system coping with a yeast overgrowth manages better with cooked vegetables rather than raw ones. If possible, however, vegetables should be eaten both raw and cooked, according to the following excellent pattern:

One of the main meals (say, lunch) every day can be a source of protein such as fish, poultry, lamb, egg or fresh nuts, together with as large a mixed salad as your imagination can conjure up and your appetite can cope with. The other main meal should also contain protein as well as cooked vegetables (steamed, baked or stir-fried).

The source of protein at each meal does not have to be based on animals. Combining a cereal and a pulse (for example, brown rice with lentils or millet with chickpeas) at the same meal ensures that adequate protein is available to the body.

What is essential is that adequate protein be eaten daily, whether from a 'safe' animal source or from the judicious mixing of complementary vegetable proteins. What is adequate for one person is not necessarily so for another. For good health, people of East Asian origin require less protein than those of northern European stock. The difference lies in the efficiency with which a person digests and absorbs what proteins are eaten. Thus, 50 g of a first-class protein daily is adequate for an East Asian whereas 75 g (or more, depending upon levels of activity) may be required by a European.[15]

Since natural live yoghurt (a good source of protein) is likely to be included in the diet, eating protein at both of the main meals in addition to yoghurt is probably not necessary. It should be possible to have, for example, a mixed salad with a jacket potato or savoury rice dish and additional nuts and seeds for one meal, while having a 'safe' animal protein with a variety of cooked vegetables for the other. In any case, the tastes and preferences of individuals differ markedly, and the variations that are possible as to what to eat are so great that no more than broad guidelines can be given.

The essential rules are:

1 Avoid all yeast-based or yeast-containing foods (unless certain that there is no sensitivity to these)
2 Avoid all sugar and refined cereal products, and foods containing them
3 Avoid all foods and drinks based on fermentation (with the possible exception of cider vinegar as discussed above)
4 Avoid meat, poultry and fish containing residues of antibiotics and steroids
5 Eat three meals daily
6 Ensure adequate protein intake
7 Ensure that a high dietary fibre content is maintained
8 Avoid fruit for the first three or four weeks of the programme.

INCREASING THE VARIETY OF FOODS

Once symptoms of Candida overgrowth begin to ease – usually after two months or so – and you find that you would like to increase the range of foods, it is permissible to experiment a bit. But this should not be before the end of the second month on the programme, and then, only if there has been a marked improvement. If you do introduce a food which has been on the 'no-go' list, observe the consequences carefully. If there are none, you may extend your experiment to another food after a week or so. But if symptoms return, go back to basic avoidance, as specified above, until they calm down again.

Such experimentation is necessary only if you feel constrained by the limitations imposed by the programme so that, at least, you introduce foods carefully with the knowledge that they might (only might) upset things. If they do, this only means that you must be patient for a little longer. There are many excellent books available which explain the principles of rotation diets to help you formulate a strategy for eating certain foods only periodically in a systematic way.[16] It is not suggested that sugar-containing foods be reintroduced at this stage other than in the very minimal sense – by perhaps introducing a little honey.

Other essential information regarding food

Moulds are present on most fruits and vegetables, and these should be well washed and eaten fresh as the longer they are kept, the more the mould development will be encouraged. Yeasts also grow on grains of all sorts, so the fresher these are, the better. Many people with Candida problems are allergic or sensitive to grains. This allergy may diminish during the programme of Candida control, and a little experimentation is in order after two or three months if your symptoms have generally declined.

A reminder is called for regarding nuts. Peanuts and pistachios, in particular, are subject to mould development (with peanuts, this is a highly toxic, potentially cancer-causing agent). All nuts, unless freshly opened by you, contain some degree of mould and certainly a degree of rancidity of the natural oils. Only eat nuts that are currently in season and freshly opened by yourself, or avoid them completely.

Apart from a little butter and natural live yoghurt, it is suggested that all milk products be avoided (Dr Truss allows cottage cheese).

If you are at a restaurant or if friends invite you for a meal, make sure that you stick to basics. Avoid sauces and gravy, desserts, stuffing and any obvious undesirables, such as mushrooms. A meat, poultry or fish dish with salad or vegetables is the safest bet, and stick to water instead of wine.

What about sugar substitutes for those who cannot keep away from sweet things? These are open to question as far as long-term safety is concerned but, in small amounts for the duration of the programme (at least six months), they at least do not encourage Candida growth. Aspartame and saccharin fall into this category, but not fructose, corn syrup or any other sugar-rich substitutes for the real thing. Instead, fructo-oligosaccharide (FOS) is somewhat sweet and not only does not encourage yeast, it feeds the friendly bacteria. It can safely be added to foods as a sweetener in as large a quantity as you wish (for best results, use not less than 8 g of FOS daily).

Remember that all commercial breakfast foods, such as corn flakes, are undesirable. They are processed and most contain yeast and/or sugar products.

Water from the tap should be filtered before drinking, if possible. There are many inexpensive water filters available that will remove a variety of organic substances which otherwise find their way into food or directly into you. Most bottled water is acceptable, but not carbonated if you have problems with bloating and gas. As for coffee and tea, these are undesirable not only as sources of mould, but because they stimulate sugar release from the liver, which feeds Candida, and increases pancreatic activity, which exhausts this vital organ further. Another good reason for not using tea is because it reduces the efficiency of both protein and iron absorption by the body, and coffee is a suspect in the development of certain kinds of cancer. Some herb teas have been found to help in the control of Candida and related problems; rooibosch, a South African tea substitute can be used by allergic subjects, and taheebo or pau d'arco (helpful in catarrh problems caused by Candida) etc., is also worth trying.

Steaming vegetables is the best way to retain the vital minerals so often destroyed and lost in boiling. Dressing a salad with lemon juice, olive oil and a little natural yoghurt can replace the vinegar or other dressings not compatible with the programme.

As the programme begins to work and symptoms become tolerable or disappear, so can a limited quantity of foods based on or containing mould or yeast be reintroduced. Wine or real ale in limited amounts, or tea and coffee may be taken occasionally. However, the need for vigilance must continue because the programme cannot remove Candida from the scene altogether. Even if the problem is attacked aggressively with the use of antifungal drugs in addition to the programme outlined above, the yeast will remain in the body.

The long-term answer after achieving control of the yeast by these means is to maintain a high level of immune function through your diet by ensuring its nutrient value as well as avoiding those factors which you now know can reduce its optimum defence capability. This does not mean that the programme is a life sentence. It is hoped that, after a while, you will come to regard sweet tastes as unpleasant and no longer crave, or even enjoy, sweet foods. It is also hoped that your new sense of wellbeing will help to motivate you towards the pattern of eating suggested here more or less permanently not only because it is good for you, but because you actually enjoy it.

Other factors

It is important to not only avoid foods and beverages containing fungal or yeast substances, but also to avoid inhaling these organisms or their spores. This is why you should keep well away from damp, dank places and deal with the presence of any mould, or wet or dry rot, in your environment. If there is any danger of damp in rooms, cupboards, cellars or lofts, do something positive to eliminate it, or, if possible, move to a new, damp-free residence. Your home could be making you ill. This advice is especially pertinent to anyone who notices a worsening of symptoms when the weather is damp or muggy, or who is obviously affected by contact with mouldy or dank environments.

LIGHT

The availability of full-spectrum light is another important element which can improve your immune system and general function.[17] It is known that the eyes contain photo-receptors, which carry impulses directly to the pituitary gland, which lies in the head. This is the 'master gland' of the body, and is vital for normal health and functioning. If the eyes are denied light (not artificial light, but the full spectrum from the sun), then demonstrable imbalances occur in the hormonal system as a direct result. Behavioural and physical symptoms can occur in consequence. The immune system is affected, and this is the reason for our concern. The advice to all who wear eyeglasses or spend most of their days indoors behind glass is that they should get outside for at least half an hour a day, with nothing between natural light and their eyes. If going out is not possible, then spend time by an open window without wearing glasses or contact lenses. In a polluted city, the light rays from the sun are distorted to some degree, and so more exposure is required. Never look directly at the sun, not even on an overcast day, as just being outdoors is enough if your eyes are not covered.

Full-spectrum fluorescent lighting units are available, and health and productivity have been found to improve dramatically when such lighting is introduced into the workplace. As an additional support for the immune system, having access to unpolluted, unfiltered, pure light is a positive step.

EXERCISE

The immune system also benefits from adequate exercise, such as trying to apply the ideals set out in Dr Kenneth Cooper's book *The New Aerobics*.[18] At least every other day, you should indulge in a form of physical exercise sufficient to stimulate the circulation and respiration. A brisk walk of one or two miles is the safest and easiest form of exercise that can produce such results. Cooper's book is recommended reading. Its beauty lies in the way it is applicable to anyone, at any stage of fitness or otherwise, so that any reader can gradually lift himself to a level of optimum fitness in slow stages.

STRESS

The avoidance of stress and anxiety is a fundamental need, as is the requirement we all have for what can be called TLC (tender loving care). These ingredients for a healthy life have been well described in many popular and easily available books. That the immune system needs such input should encourage the study of relaxation and meditation as well as stress-reducing methods in general. I have outlined a programme of stress-reduction in my book *Stress*,[19] which should be helpful in both assessing and dealing with those stress factors which affect quality of life.

SEX

Considering the overall importance of the immune system, it is worth commenting on an area of research which tends to be ignored because of its unpopular message. There is abundant proof that women who have sexual relations with a large number of men are more prone to cancer of the womb than those who have relations with only one or a few partners.[15] Early sexual experience is also known to predispose the individual to diseases which should be prevented by a healthy immune system. Candida is highly contagious when skin contact is involved, especially if this includes abrasion and tissue irritation.

HIV is more common among homosexuals who have multiple partners than among those who have steady relationships with a single partner. It would seem, therefore, that there is a role for the immune system in any close physical (sexual) contact. If the immune system is called upon to cope with antigens from a wide variety of different sources (and sperm cells are foreign proteins to a woman's body), then this may well be a factor in depleting a person's immune response (along with a great number of other factors).

This viewpoint has been expressed in numerous medical journals since the AIDS epidemic began,[20, 21] and points to relative sexual fidelity as being desirable for anyone who wishes to maintain an intact immune system. This does not mean that celibacy is called for, but that frequent changes in sexual partners are best avoided – whether heterosexual or homosexual – at the very least during the anti-Candida programme.

NOTE

It should be clear from the information provided in earlier chapters of this book that no antibiotics, steroids or contraceptive pills should be used during the course of the anti-Candida programme unless absolutely vital.

REFERENCES

1 Bodey G, Fainstein V (eds). 'Candidiasis in the gastrointestinal tract', *Candidiasis*, New York: Raven Press, 1985
2 Bolivar R *et al*. 'Candidiasis of the gastrointestinal tract', *Candidiasis*, New York: Raven Press, 1985
3 Rubinstein E *et al*. 'Antibacterial activity of the pancreatic fluid', *Gastroenterology* 1985; 88: 927–32
4 Jorgensen B. 'Baker's yeast allergy in candidiasis patients', *J Adv Med* 1994; 7(1): 43–9

5 Truss C. *The Missing Diagnosis*, Birmingham, AL: Self-published, 1980
6 Werbach M. *Nutritional Influences on Illness* [Suppl], Tarzana, CA: Third Line Press, 1991: S13
7 Gutierrez J *et al.* 'Circulating Candida antigens and antibodies: useful markers of candidemia', *J Clin Microbiol* 1993; 31(9)
8 Brown & Binkley. *Yeast: A Brief Description of Common Sources*, 1980
9 Personal communication with Dr C. Orian Truss, 1983
10 Crook W. *The Yeast Connection*, Jackson, TN: Professional Books, 1988
11 Horowitz B *et al.* 'Sugar chromatography studies in recurrent Candida vulvovaginitis', *J Reprod Med* 1984; 29(7): 441–3
12 'Less sugar/vaginal candidiasis', *Fam Pract News* 1999; 29(23): 21
13 Samarayanake L *et al.* 'Proteolytic potential of *Candida albicans* in human saliva supplemented by glucose', *J Med Microbiol* 1984; 17(1): 13–22
14 Bland J. 'Candida albicans: an alternative therapy for an unexpected problem', *J Alt Med* 1983; July: 18–19
15 Bland J (ed). *Medical Application of Clinical Nutrition*, New Canaan, CN: Keats Publishing, 1983
16 Forman R. *How to Control Your Allergies*, London: Larchmont Books, 1979
17 Ott J. *Light Radiation and You*, Devin Adair, 1982
18 Cooper K. *The New Aerobics*, New York: Bantam, 1977
19 Chaitow L. *Stress*, Wellingborough, Northants: Thorsons, 1984
20 Editorial, *N Engl J Med* 1981; 10 Dec
21 Editorial, *Lancet* 1981; 12 Dec

7 | *Putting your anti-Candida programme together*

To get a strong indication as to whether *Candida albicans* overgrowth is a feature of your health problems, carefully answer the questionnaire in Chapter 4.

The following suggestions do not take account of every possible variation, but offer a guide to what is likely to be successful in controlling Candida in most instances.

The strongest recommendation is that you consult an expert in the treatment of yeast problems. It is best to find a local expert who is either a naturopathic practitioner with sound qualifications, a nutritionally trained medical practitioner (such as a clinical ecologist), a homoeopath who uses nutritional methods, a well-qualified nutritionist, or some other healthcare professional with the appropriate knowledge and experience (many chiropractors and osteopaths will also have studied nutritional therapies). If in doubt, ask for details of their qualifications and experience (*see also Resources, pages 173–4*).

If economic factors or a lack of an expert practitioner in your area result in your decision to try self-treatment, I urge you not to pick and choose only those aspects you feel you want to try, but to follow comprehensively all elements of the anti-Candida programme, as described in previous chapters and summarized here:

- antifungal methods
- detoxification plus liver and immune support
- repopulation with probiotic organisms

- a basic anti-Candida diet plus prebiotics
- use of additional and local treatment methods as indicated (such as healing the mucous membrane in a 'leaky gut').

Keeping track of symptoms

You should list your major symptoms on the left-hand side of a sheet of paper; underline each one and extend that line clear across the page. Then, draw columns (vertical lines down the page) to divide the page into a series of 'boxes' into which, every day, next to each symptom you enter a score reflecting the symptom's intensity over the past 24 hours.

At the top of each column, enter the date and, next to the symptom, enter a score value – for example, you may decide on a range of 0 to 3, with 0 for no symptoms at all to 3 being the worst your thrush irritation can ever be. You can do this with all the other symptoms, such as indigestion, fatigue, headache, muscle pain and so on.

The very bottom of the page – say the last inch or so – should be left open so that, under the appropriate date, you can enter a total symptom score (all your individual scores added up for that day) as well as any short notes to remind you of any special factors, such as 'started acidophilus', 'period started', 'caught a cold', 'ran out of oregano oil capsules' – anything that will jog your memory when you look back at the score sheet weeks or months later as to what factors influenced the scores on that day.

You should keep the score sheet handy (on the refrigerator held by a magnet perhaps) and fill it in at the same time each day, say, just before your evening meal or at bedtime.

The value of this is enormous since, as you make changes in your programme, you can judge their impact on

symptom	date	date	date	date	date	date	date	date	date	date	date
Tired	3	3	3	2	2	1	2	1	1	2	1
Gas	3	3	3	2	2	2	0	1	1	2	1
Head	1	1	2	1	3	2	3	1	1	1	1
Runs	1	1	3	3	1	0	1	0	0	2	0
Skin-itch	1	0	0	0	3	0	1	1	1	1	0
PMT	3	3	3	2	2	1	1	0	0	1	0
Sore mouth	2	2	2	2	1	1	1	2	1	1	0
Other	?	?	?	?	?	?	?	?	?	?	?
Other	?	?	?	?	?	?	?	?	?	?	?
Total	14	13	16	12	14	7	9	6	10	3	
Note		start programme							period began		

your individual symptoms as well as on your total score. This helps to unravel the sometimes complicated causes of your problems. For example, you may have five or six symptoms listed, but only three of these may have changed markedly within the first few months of the programme. This tells you that the symptoms which improved were probably directly related to your Candida overgrowth, while the other symptoms were not and, therefore, require some other form of attention.

It is also useful to remind yourself of where you have been in terms of symptom intensity as the weeks go by. A satisfactory slow decline of scores is very gratifying (with minor ups and downs, which can occur for many reasons). It is also useful to know if scores are *not* declining, as this may be an alarm signal that either the problem is not Candida-related at all or the programme is inadequate. In either case, it is better to be aware of this sooner rather than later.

SYMPTOM SCORE SHEET

The example score sheet shows how you can keep track of symptoms and the individual aspects of the programme as they affect your health.

Do not expect major beneficial changes within two months of starting the programme if your condition is severe, and you should also anticipate that, for a couple of weeks, your scores could increase at first, as yeast die-off occurs and the detoxification process begins.

Since the comprehensive antifungal programme presented here calls for a great many changes and all of these are potentially stressful, to allow your body to 'get used to' the changes, it is best to introduce them in stages – first eliminating allergens, then reducing and cutting out sugars, then introducing immune-enhancing nutrients and herbs, then starting the liver-support strategies, and the pre- and probiotic programme followed by the antifungal methods.

This can take several weeks to get into place and you should expect that some odd symptoms may appear during this time, especially in terms of altered bowel function, abdominal 'noises' and, very likely, nausea and or headache/fatigue in excess of what you have previously noted. These changes indicate the onset of the detoxification process and should not be cause for anxiety – and certainly should not stop you from persisting with the programme. This is where expert support and advice are particularly useful, especially if you are trying to introduce these changes single-handedly without the emotional and practical support that is so helpful during such changes.

A *10-point strategy*

First, reduce as much as possible, or stop using completely (after consulting your medical adviser), any steroid medication and antibiotics. Then:

1 If you regularly suffer from 'indigestion', dyspepsia, heartburn, 'acid stomach' or bloating, consider the methods outlined in Chapter 6 regarding supplementation with betaine hydrochloride or Swedish bitters to see whether these problems are not, in fact, due to an inadequate acid supply.

2 If you have allergic/sensitivity-type symptoms, introduce a broad-spectrum enzyme supplement with each main meal and assess the benefits over a period of several weeks.

3 If you are sensitive to yeast-type foods, eliminate these (as per the lists in Chapter 6) for at least two, and ideally three, months before attempting a challenge

and possible 'rotation' of the foods involved. If you are aware of dairy or wheat allergies, eliminate these foods altogether for the first three months of the programme before reassessing their impact.

4 Eliminate sugar and refined carbohydrates (*see Chapter 6*).

5 Introduce immune-enhancing supplementation and liver-support herbs (*see Chapter 5*).

6 After introducing all of the above as appropriate to your condition, all the while assessing your symptom scores (*see above*), begin incorporating these other elements of the diet:
   - introduce pre- and probiotic supplementation (*see Chapter 5*), and anticipate some additional bloating at first
   - introduce antifungal strategies (*see Chapter 5*), choosing one or two of the listed products and ensuring the highest quality possible (*see pages 173–4* for contact details for The Nutri Centre, from where all the products mentioned in this book can be ordered for postal delivery if you do not have an easily accessible local health store to advise and supply you)
   - introduce methods to reduce bowel permeability (*see Chapter 5*) if there are symptoms indicating bowel irritation (such as food sensitivities and/or a previous diagnosis of IBS and/or mucus in the bowel movements and/or a longstanding or severe degree of yeast involvement)
   - introduce local measures to treat any local signs of yeast involvement in the mouth or vagina, for example (*see Chapter 5*).

7 If yeast die-off is severe, there are strategies for reducing the toxic load, using herbal and nutritional methods (nutrients such as molybdenum and zinc, or the amino acids L-cysteine or L-methionine and/or L-carnitine) as well as herbal liver support, such as silymarin (milk thistle extract) and/or ginger.

8 Introduce detoxification methods which are not diet-related, such as skin-brushing, Epsom salts baths, various aromatherapy essential oil baths, and also consider relaxation, breathing retraining, yoga and other stress-reducing, immune-enhancing methods.

9 If bowel dysbiosis (chronic bowel stasis, for example) is causing increased toxicity, colonic irrigation may be useful at this time as may the use of 'coffee enemas'. As these need to be individually prescribed according to need, no details are given in this text as it would be unwise to experiment with such methods without professional guidance.

10 After two months, a change in the programme may be called for, such as the introduction of modified antifungal strategies, depending on your progress so far. Changes in your diet may also be permissible if sensitivities are reduced.

Details of these 10 points are outlined in Chapters 5 and 6 but, because individual features and factors apply in every case of Candida overgrowth, it is impossible to give specific details to suit all needs.

If your symptom scores are declining steadily (albeit with ups and downs due to particular circumstances), there is every reason to press on. If symptoms are not markedly improved after two months of consistent application of the main elements of the programme, it is time to reassess your condition and how you are dealing with it. At such a time, expert advice is probably called for.

How often are you likely to need to consult anyone for advice?

Certainly, you should consult a professional once at the beginning of the programme, and probably at six- to eight-week intervals during the following three- to six-month course. In severe cases, the programme may need to be maintained for up to a year.

If special needs call for more frequent consultations or treatments, this should be established at the very beginning of the course. Nowadays, once the programme is underway, it is possible to advise patients via e-mail where minor fine-tuning of the programme is needed, thus avoiding the need for face-to-face consultations.

A maintenance programme is usually called for when Candida is under control – you need to maintain a low-sugar, low-fat diet with wholesome, nutritious and balanced food forming the major elements of the diet. At this time, some relaxation of the restrictions is usually possible and the intake of nutrients can usually be reduced to only probiotic supplementation and perhaps a multivitamin/mineral nutrient support capsule/tablet daily.

Many thousands of people have benefited from following the advice given in this book. Although it may not take the place of individually prescribed methods that take account of your individual needs, it is nevertheless a useful starting point if you have found yourself unable to get help from your usual health advisers. Hopefully, as ever more GPs become aware of the value of such an approach, you will find support within the National Health Service. Until then, there is a need for you to take responsibility, to take action and, if possible, to take advice.

The final chapter of this book presents a selection of case histories which may be of value to you in evaluating similarities with your own condition.

8 | *Case histories*

This chapter includes a number of case histories where people who either had a yeast overgrowth, or thought they did, are described. The features which emerge as common, and the differences, are emphasized, and you should be able to identify with aspects of at least some of the problems, treatment and health outcomes of these individuals.

Care has been taken to disguise the individuals in each case history by altering significant facts so that they remain anonymous. Such changes have not, however, altered the medical facts, which remain as a testament to the effectiveness of an anti-Candida approach to a variety of health problems when the symptoms are caused, or are at least significantly affected, by yeast overgrowth.

A number of the cases here involve men, which serves to emphasize that yeast overgrowth is not just a women's problem (although, by far, the majority of cases of candidiasis involve women).

Case 1: AC, male, age 49

Mr C is a recovering heroin addict and alcoholic (he has been 'clean' for 18 months). He presented himself for advice and treatment with a long list of symptoms, including chronic fatigue, headaches, nausea, digestive distress (bloating, indigestion, intermittent diarrhoea), skin irritation, itchy anus and athlete's foot as well as sleep disturbance, muscular and joint pain, anxiety and panic attacks. He reported that he had been sent to hospital for his symptoms, and had been given a diagnosis of moderate cirrhosis of the liver as well as a hepatitis C infection.

He was already receiving regular acupuncture, counselling and reflexology via a support group accessed through social services and felt that these were all helpful, and had been referred by his GP for nutritional and herbal advice in the hope that his digestion would be improved, despite already having seen a dietitian who had directed him toward a more balanced eating pattern in which his sugar intake had been severely cut. He was, he said, trying to stick to the new high-protein, high-complex carbohydrate (such as vegetables and grains), low-simple carbohydrate diet. When he followed this advice, he noticed that many of his symptoms were indeed eased, but the bloating, diarrhoea, itching and fatigue remained almost daily events.

A careful look at his medical history revealed that he had had multiple antibiotic courses over the past 20 years and that his diet for much of that time had been very poor, with simple carbohydrates as his main food source (sugars, fats and, of course, alcohol). He was aware that his digestive symptoms were aggravated when he consumed sugary foods.

Yeast overgrowth (Candida) was clearly a part of his complicated medical condition and, after some discussion, he agreed that we should focus on three strategies:

1 Improve the ecology of his digestive tract to remove as much stress as possible on his already damaged liver and to encourage an improved nutritional status. As part of this process, a gentle detoxification programme was to be followed, including both liver support and anti-Candida protocols.

2 A programme of graduated exercise (toning, stretching and aerobic) as well as breathing retraining would be followed to gradually regain a degree of physical fitness.

3 Emotional support would be encouraged alongside the counselling he was already receiving in the form of relaxation and meditation exercises, particularly autogenic training.

A periodic monodiet (a rice-only diet) was suggested for 36 hours every two weeks for three months (1 kg of rice, cooked and eaten in small portions throughout the day, and not less than 2 litres of water daily) to enhance detoxification. A combination of dandelion extract, artichoke and milk thistle (*Silybum marianum*) was recommended to support liver function as well as reduced glutathione (100 mg daily).

Anti-Candida measures included the use of Horopeito/ Mikoplex together with a daily supplement of probiotic organisms, and prebiotic FOS (fructo-oligosaccharides) – 8 g daily in divided doses. The mucous membrane of the digestive tract was allowed to heal by means of a herbal/nutrient combination containing L-glutamine, slippery elm, marshmallow and liquorice (*Glycyrrhiza glabra*)[1] – taken between meals. General nutritional support was suggested with an advanced antioxidant formulation (vitamins A and C, selenium, L-cysteine, a multivitamin/ mineral supplement and biotin).

The general dietary advice was for a high-protein (low-fat), high-fibre (low-sugar) lacto-ovo vegetarian diet, which included abundant vegetables (cooked rather than raw for ease of digestion). He was asked to drink not less than 2 litres of water daily.

He was taught a calming antiarousal breathing pattern[2] to help reduce anxiety symptoms; the exercises were both described and demonstrated.

After a shaky start (die-off period) when his headaches and general malaise were worse for two weeks, a gradual but eventually marked degree of improvement emerged over a four-month period (with several brief and minor setbacks along the way), with better digestion, fewer headaches, enhanced sleep, reduced anxiety and more energy. By the end of the third month, he had no signs of athlete's foot or anal itching and, in his own words, he felt 'close to normal'.

He has been asked to repeat the 'rice detox' once a month indefinitely after reporting an enormous degree of energy enhancement and sense of wellbeing for several days after each monodiet period. He has also been advised to continue the probiotic and prebiotic strategies and liver support, but the antifungal herbs were stopped after five months.

This was a case of a severely compromised individual who diligently stuck to his programme after years of self-neglect. His health has been permanently compromised, but his yeast-related conditions have been eliminated and his general health improved. His underlying liver condition remains the same and will require caution for the rest of his life.

Case 2: BB, male, age 35

This pleasant young man consulted me for his irritable bowel (IBS) condition, although his most pressing health concern involved moderately severe ankylosing spondylitis (AS or 'bamboo spine', which results in gradual fusion of the spinal joints into a forward-curved state). The AS had become evident in his early 20s, starting with low back and pelvic pain. He was already somewhat stooped and received regular physiotherapy to help maintain mobility, but was in considerable discomfort as he had to force his neck into a marked degree of backward bending just to be able to see where he was going. Apart from anti-inflammatory and painkilling medication (which aggravated his bowel problems), he was not receiving any medical attention for either the IBS or the AS.

Careful questioning elicited the information that he also suffered from skin irritation (groin, underarms, feet), and experienced periodic episodes of ringworm and athlete's foot.

In his teens and early 20s, he had undergone a lengthy course of antibiotics for acne, and thought that this was when his IBS had started. These symptoms were typical, involving almost constant bloating, some indigestion and diarrhoea several times daily, interspersed with periodic episodes of severe constipation. A stool analysis revealed what organisms were active in his digestive tract – both *Klebsiella* (a bacteria) and Candida overgrowth were found.

Research by A. Ebringer in the mid-1980s[3] had shown that, when the normal flora of the intestines are damaged (possibly by excessive antibiotic use), *Klebsiella* overgrowth can develop. These bacteria can provoke an autoimmune response in people with a genetic predisposition. Ebringer concluded that people with a particular tissue type represented 98 per cent of those with AS, which largely affects men and usually when they are young. Ebringer stated: '*Klebsiella* thrives on a diet rich in starch (carbohydrates). If you cut out starchy carbohydrates such as rice, potatoes and refined flour products, then you reduce the number of *Klebsiella* in the gut, and subsequently the production of antibodies to the bacteria which cause the inflammation' (as reported in *The Independent*).

The protocol of treatment, which Mr B agreed to follow, included an anti-Candida approach with dietary strategies that Ebringer had formulated to diminish *Klebsiella* activity. Mr B was advised to eliminate bread, pasta and cereals of all sorts, rice and potatoes as well as sugary foods. There was no restriction on vegetables, fruit, eggs, cheese and fish.

His anti-Candida programme included high doses of quality probiotics (*Lactobacillus acidophilus* and *Bifidobacterium*) to encourage repopulation of the gut, 8 g daily of FOS (prebiotics), a herbal combination of *Echinacea*, *Hydrastis* and berberine to remove both Candida and *Klebsiella*, and general nutritional support from high-quality multivitamin/mineral sources.

Because the bowel was so compromised and as Mr B was somewhat underweight, a supplement based on bluegreen algae (rich in protein) was advised several times daily, away from regular mealtimes. This was taken as a drink (soy or rice milk) into which the powdered algae were stirred.

Over a nine-month period, the severity of all his symptoms declined markedly, as evidenced by a reduced requirement for analgesic and anti-inflammatory medications. Pain was reduced and no additional spinal restriction was apparent, both of which were symptoms that had been progressively worsening prior to the dietary changes.

IBS was gradually improved so that bloating became unusual, indigestion almost never happened and explosive, loose, watery bowel movements only occurred once or twice a week instead of several times daily. A follow-up stool analysis showed very low levels of bacteria and yeast, calling for at least another six to nine months on the programme before, hopefully, none would be found and the programme could be slowly stopped (although the basic dietary strategy should be followed indefinitely).

Case 3: HS, female, age 40

The details of this case history are given in greater depth than others in this chapter as this example is so typical of the many women who struggle through life with a host of symptoms, many of them Candida-related. HS is one of those described by American researcher Jeffrey Bland as being 'vertically ill' – not sick enough to lie down ('horizontally ill'!), but with a range of minor problems which, together, made her life a constant battle.

This pleasant woman, a retail fashion-store manager, consulted me with the following symptoms (listed in the order of importance she attached to them at the time), which were current and had been present for approximately three years:

- Fluctuating (sometimes extreme) fatigue, worse in the early morning, late morning and mid-afternoon
- Associated difficulties in concentration and short-term memory, coinciding with the fatigue fluctuation ('brain fog')
- Mood swings and an increasing sense of anxiety; a recent panic attack when out shopping
- Widespread muscular pain, mainly in the neck, shoulders, arms, chest and low back (plus morning stiffness), which she described as a 'deep ache', but sometimes 'sharp' or 'burning'
- An oppressive 'heavy weight' on her chest and an inability to breathe deeply
- Irritable bowel, abdominal bloating (more or less constant), tendency to constipation, rare episodes of diarrhoea (her GP diagnosed IBS)
- Poor sleep pattern; wakes frequently, dreams a lot
- Recent steady weight gain, now about 7 kg above ideal weight, she thinks
- Increasing sensitivity to cold, bright light, loud noise
- Premenstrual symptoms (increased fatigue and mood swings, fluid retention, sugar cravings, 'terrible headaches')
- Dry skin, fungal-infected toenails

- Periodic thrush (usually coinciding with her menstrual cycle), both vaginal and oral, as well as anal itch (more persistent than other fungal symptoms)
- Loss of interest in sexual activity (she is in a long-term, stable relationship).

All of her symptoms were worse after alcohol and sugar-rich food, and she reacted badly (with extreme fatigue) to foods containing yeast.

HISTORY

Her early history revealed a happy and stable childhood. One sister (she has two) has 'multiple allergies', the other is 'fine'. As a child, HS had persistent ear, nose and throat infections involving multiple courses of antibiotics. Tonsils and adenoids were removed at age 12. She had severe acne from age 15 onwards and eventual antibiotic treatment for 6 months at age 17. She started taking the contraceptive pill at age 19, and had taken this 'on and off' for 10 years. She married at age 22 and earned a degree in business studies at 23. There was a termination at 24 and she was divorced at age 25. At the time of consultation, she had been in a stable relationship for the past 10 years, but there were no children and, as a couple, she said they had no wish for any.

She worked in a highly competitive and stressful work environment, managing a staff of eight, with her employers constantly setting turnover and profit targets.

She believed that her current health problems followed a holiday in Spain, some four years previously, where she developed gastroenteritis that was treated locally with a course of antibiotics, followed by a repeat course on her return to the UK; the digestive problems recurred within a week. She acknowledged a tendency to constipation, bloating and indigestion as well as having had PMS and recurrent thrush since her teens, but these all worsened dramatically during the year following the Spanish incident. She was very worried that her 'brain fog' and lack of energy was impairing her performance at work (which despite 'stress', she enjoyed) and that she might lose her well-paid job. She also worried about her personal relationship, and the effect her lack of sexual interest and general lethargy was having on it.

INTERVENTIONS

Her GP had been generally supportive but unhelpful, telling HS that there was nothing significantly wrong with her, medically speaking. The GP had prescribed various anti-fungals (systemic and topical) which had given short-term help to the thrush and skin problems. The subject of depression was discussed, but neither the GP nor the patient believed this to be a factor. Nevertheless, the patient had self-prescribed a course of St John's wort 'just in case', with no significant benefit. On the recommendation of a friend, she had attended a Traditional Chinese Medicine clinic and had taken a selection of 'foul-smelling' herbs for some months, with some benefit to her digestive system, her pre-menstrual symptoms and her dry skin, but she eventually gave this up because of the bother of preparing the herbal brew.

To use her own words, she was 'at her wit's end', and very anxious, which was exhausting her and making her sleep pattern even worse. There was nothing clinically significant noted at the first consultation in her cardiac function or blood pressure, although she seemed to slightly hyperventilate and to be very tense.

DIET AT CONSULTATION

Her dietary pattern was:

- Breakfast (7.30 am): one or two cups coffee (always black with one sugar) or (weekends) egg, bacon, toast and coffee, or cereal (Special K) and milk

- Mid-morning (10.30 am): coffee, doughnut or biscuit
- Lunch (1.00 pm): sandwich (tuna, ham, cheese) and coffee
- Mid-afternoon (3.30 pm): tea or coffee and biscuit
- Evening (6.30–9.00 pm): if eating out (two or three times a week), Chinese, Indian or Italian (pasta/pizza), dessert, coffee plus wine (two or three glasses) and, once a week, vodka (one or two); if eating at home, most likely a convenience meal with one or two vegetables or salad, or a fish & chips takeaway plus wine and coffee

Salads and cooked vegetables play a small part in the diet; fruit intake was minimal. Coffee intake was 6–8 cups/day; water intake was around 0.5 litres a day. She took a multi-vitamin/mineral supplement and sometimes vitamin C; her pre-period sugar cravings resulted in consumption of several bars of chocolate daily for a week or so (sometimes more); she consciously avoided dairy foods because she believed they made her digestion even worse than it was already; she reported increased bloating after sugar and wine.

RECOMMENDATIONS

In deciding what to recommend, the fluctuating nature of her fatigue and muscle pain strongly suggested environ-mental (probably dietary) intolerances or sensitivities. Her hypoglycaemic symptoms (periodic energy crashes) needed to be balanced by changes in her eating pattern in terms of both timing and content. Her weight gain, fatigue and dry skin were all suggestive of an underactive thyroid condi-tion, which called for investigation and could be linked to the allergies she was experiencing. Her 'tight chest' and anxiety (and panic) symptoms almost certainly were related to a pattern of upper-chest breathing, which should be relatively easy to correct if she was prepared to practise spe-cific breathing-retraining exercises. Such breathing patterns (which can alter blood chemistry, making it too alkaline due to excessive loss of carbon dioxide) when combined with hypoglycaemia can produce dramatically severe symptoms, particularly during the progesterone (premenstrual) phase of the cycle. These changes in blood chemistry can also make allergic reactions more severe because of heightened levels of histamine.

Her antibiotic and steroid (contraceptive pill) history suggested ways in which her bowel ecology had been compromised, and her fungal and IBS history supported this likelihood. Fungal overgrowth could account for her bowel (and thrush) symptoms, predisposing towards irritation and increased permeability of the mucous lining of the intestines, so allowing large molecules to cross into the bloodstream, loading the liver with increased detoxification tasks and triggering her 'intolerance' reactions. These could easily produce many of the symptoms she complained of, including fatigue and muscle pain. Her yeast sensitivity was just one more confirming feature of a yeast overgrowth. So, it seemed to me that the digestive system and 'leaky gut' should receive the primary attention, with probiotic supplementation, anti-Candida herbs and exclusion strategies to reduce her intolerance reactions.

Recommended changes included:

- Decreased caffeine intake (gradual) leading to complete elimination over a period of four to six weeks
- Elimination of all alcohol intake
- Increased water intake to 2.5 litres daily
- More desirable food choices (increased protein and complex carbohydrates, reduced simple carbohydrates and, as far as possible, avoidance of anything fermented or containing yeast (basically an anti-Candida diet).

She was encouraged to eat five or six small meals daily, with a relatively high proportion of protein. If this was 'difficult' because of work pressure, a protein supplement ('full-spectrum amino acids') should be taken on rising/mid-morning/mid-afternoon and before bedtime. I suggested that she take 200 mcg of Glucose Tolerance Factor (chromium) daily to assist in stabilizing blood sugar levels. This frequently improves fatigue as well as reducing craving tendencies. Various other supplements were suggested, including calcium and magnesium, flaxseed oil, zinc and a multivitamin/mineral supplement.

She was advised to follow a comprehensive antifungal protocol for at least three, and ideally six, months, including pre- and probiotics, antifungal herbs, bowel-soothing herbs to reduce gut permeability and liver-support herbs. I suggested that an investigation of thyroid function might be delayed until the benefits of the anti-Candida diet became apparent, probably within three months. The possible benefits of periodic short-term fasting were explained as an option (36–48 hours every two weeks on water). Relaxation, meditation and autogenic training methods were taught for home application, and aerobic activity was encouraged within her current limitations, together with yoga-type stretching (or Pilates). She was asked to maintain a daily symptom score sheet as a means of monitoring the influence of the therapeutic strategies.

A further consultation for review of progress was advised after four weeks, with a strong suggestion that the restoration of a reasonable degree of health would take anything from three to six months, and possibly longer.

OUTCOME
At four months, after some ups and downs of her symptoms during the first six weeks, the following changes were reported:

- Energy levels were at least 75 per cent better, and brain fog was virtually 100 per cent better

- Sleep was more normal, but still patchy when work pressure was heavy
- Aches and pains had eased by approximately 50 per cent, and were much better for some hours after her regular (daily at home, once a week at a class) yoga sessions
- Thrush and PMS were dramatically better
- Mood swings were largely a thing of the past
- IBS only reappeared for a few days before her periods, and then only if she was careless with her diet.

Her most persistent symptoms at four months were:

- Skin, which still had some fungal patches
- Weight, which she considered was still a little above her ideal, despite having lost 4 kg (8.8 lb)
- As yet her libido had not shown much improvement.
- As her 'thyroid' symptoms had largely vanished no further investigation was considered necessary.
- At 12 months all her symptoms were improved including the skin, she remained sensitive to yeast-based foods (bowel reactions, plus a return of some fatigue, if she had more than one exposure to such foods within a few days of each other) and so strictly avoided these. Her weight was close to her ideal, and her libido was more normal

Case 4: SM, female, aged 42

When she arrived for her first consultation in October 1991, SM was accompanied by her husband but, as she looked so washed-out and aged beyond her years, I took him to be her son. Her hair was lank, and she was overweight and looked 'crumpled'. Her symptoms included a range of digestive complaints (intermittent diarrhoea/constipation, bloating, dyspepsia), various PMS symptoms, extreme fatigue, skin rashes especially under the breasts, which had been diagnosed as yeast-related, disturbed sleep with night sweats and extreme restlessness, depression and, of course, vaginitis and thrush. She had had these symptoms for about 15 years, ever since she had started bearing children (three so far). She was taking antidepressant medication from her GP (and had been for over a year), who supported her consulting me for her Candida problems.

She was in despair over her condition, and the fact that she was unable to be a 'good wife and mother', the role she had chosen for herself. The programme I suggested was a strict application of antifungal strategies (low sugar, low fat, abundant complex carbohydrates such as vegetables and whole grains) as well as a low-yeast pattern of eating (she had a history of sensitivity to yeast-based foods). I advised local application of *Aloe vera* juice alternating with diluted tea tree oil on the infected skin areas.

Specifically, she was prescribed a high-quality acidophilus and bifidobacteria supplement with caprylic acid and garlic capsules three times daily. A range of immune-supporting nutrients was also suggested. She kept a detailed symptom score sheet (*see Chapter 7*) and, over the next six months, her total and individual symptom scores progressively declined after the initial 10 days when, she said, 'I thought I was dying', so severe were her symptoms (nausea, headaches, lethargy, restlessness, flu-like aches). She phoned me during this yeast die-off period, and I suggested that she increase her intake of probiotics temporarily (bifidobacteria help with liver decongestion) and cut her Mycopryl dose until these symptoms lessened after a few days, at which time the programme was resumed.

After three months when I again saw her, she was significantly better, although there had been a period of about two weeks during the second month when her symptoms flared again for no apparent reason. She now looked years younger, had lost a stone (6 kg; 14 lb) without any specific effort to do so and had regained some energy.

The programme was maintained, unmodified for a further three months, by which time her symptoms had virtually disappeared. Her weight loss was now over two stone (12 kg; 28 lb), her vitality was restored, her skin clear and her bowel function normal. She asked me about stopping her antidepressant medication and I suggested she talk to her GP. However, I did write to him to say that I believed that her depression had been the result of her state of health and that she could probably be weaned off the drugs if he agreed. When I saw her for the fourth and last time after nine months (July 1992), she had a symptom score sheet ranging between '1' and '0' (compared with high 20s for 11 symptoms at the start; the 1 score was because of a periodically furred tongue). Her weight had dropped over three stone (18 kg; 42 lb) and she had successfully stopped her antidepressant medication. Her husband (who now looked older than she did!) was delighted, as were their children, and she informed me: 'They were glad to have their Mum back again.'

It was at this time that we relaxed her dietary pattern to allow a few treats of the sugary kind and her last report, by post, a year later indicated that all remained well.

SM's case well illustrates the multisymptomatic pattern that many Candida sufferers endure, the possibility that antidepressants can be prescribed for a symptom and not a cause, and the way in which a dedicated individual can put herself together again.

Case 5: FS, male, aged 34

This young gay man, who had been HIV-positive for around five years, came to see me with a single complaint –

Candida overgrowth in his mouth so severe that the tongue and cheeks were covered in white patches. It is well known that with immune suppression comes yeast activity, and a manifestation of oral thrush of this sort is extremely common among HIV-positive individuals and those with other immune-related illnesses. For the past few months, FS had started following a sound health-enhancing diet, which had previously been excessively sugar-orientated. He was, however, skipping meals from time to time due to work pressure and, on such days, his energy levels were depleted dramatically.

He was troubled with intermittent diarrhoea and was very prone to infections, with colds and chest infections almost every month, and his energy levels were lower than he felt was acceptable, making his work (in administration) an effort. Clearly, this was a condition which required careful evaluation as to how to help his immune system function more efficiently. It is unwise to 'boost' the immune system where HIV is concerned since there is evidence that aspects of the already depleted immune function are commonly overworking in an effort to maintain control of the viral infection. Instead, a modulation of immune function is called for, using selected nutrients and herbs along with an aggressive attempt at restoring bowel integrity with probiotic supplementation. His diet was tidied up (*see Chapter 6*) and a pattern of regular meals ('little and often') instituted.

A combination of supplementation with specific herbs and nutrients indicated for HIV-positive individuals plus probiotics (including *Lactobacillus bulgaricus*), herbal antifungal treatment with *Echinacea*, *Aloe vera*[1] and Tanoral mouthwash and gargle, as well as a general approach to bowel overgrowth of yeast (which must be tackled if oral thrush is to be controlled) has, over a period of 18 months, kept the yeast to only a mild degree of activity in this young man's mouth. His energy levels are increased, his ability to cope with stress is enhanced and the frequency of

1fections has reduced to once or twice a year – a
l. Seven years after his initial diagnosis, he con-
ork and live a productive life with no health
___, apart from a mild degree of yeast activity in the
mouth when he is excessively stressed at work. He has
joined a support group, has regular massage supplied free by
a leading AIDS charity in London, and practises relaxation,
meditation and yoga – and safe sex.

Case 6: SA, female, age 39 (together with Robert, aged two months)

This woman was in the early stages of pregnancy when I
first saw her. She had a history of thrush going back many
years – to her teens – when she had been prescribed antibiotics for acne. Subsequent episodes of cystitis, treated with
more antibiotics, and a lengthy spell on the Pill, had rein-
forced the condition to the point where it was more or less
permanent. The only variations were that, from time to
time, it was even worse than the usual degree of irritation,
discharge and itching. Medical attention produced no more
than short periods of relative ease – days rather than weeks
– and she had virtually abandoned discussing the problem
with her GP.

She consulted me because of her anxiety over the potential ill-effects of yeast infection on her baby. It is well
known that, during pregnancy, yeast has an easier time
in its activities due to hormonal changes. However, there
are fewer options open to treating Candida during pregnancy because of the justifiable concern for the embryo's
health. After careful evaluation of her diet, it was clear that
she was consuming excessive sugar-rich food, and this
was modified in the process of prescribing a balanced and
nutritious diet.

Supplementation with garlic and probiotics (acidophilus, bifidobacteria and *L. bulgaricus*) is perfectly safe during pregnancy, and these were all suggested according to the guidelines given in Chapter 5. I also suggested local applications of yoghurt into which acidophilus powder had been mixed, douching with *Aloe vera* in water and non-drug pessaries (*Calendula*, for example). The objective was to contain the condition until natural controls were once again able to exert themselves after pregnancy.

These tactics allowed SA a more comfortable pregnancy and a safe delivery, after which her yeast activity declined to a level that was significantly better than before her pregnancy. Unfortunately, though, within a few months of birth, her baby was suffering from both cradle cap – a yeast infection of the scalp – and nappy rash, so he, too, was brought along for advice.

By keeping the baby dry (changing nappies more frequently than usual) as well as the frequent application of a talc which contained undecylenic acid, and *Calendula* cream and/or a paste made from acidophilus and yoghurt for irritated skin patches, the external manifestations of nappy rash were kept under control while internal probiotic methods were initiated. The baby had regrettably not been able to breastfeed, so an infant formula probiotic was prescribed (containing *Bifidobacterium infantis*) along with a low-sugar diet. It was suggested that fruit juices be provided rarely and, even then, only in diluted form.

Cradle cap is a scaly skin problem which affects many infants. It is a form of seborrhoeic dermatitis and often involves Candida as well – especially if the symptoms include red bumps, pimples or pustules. The various antifungal methods suggested for local application can usually control this problem. Use of diluted tea tree oil, as found in BioCare's Dermasorb ointment, or *Aloe vera* juice or acidophilus paste will all help as long as the internal imbalances are also being dealt with (probiotic supplementation and a low-sugar diet).

The outcome for the baby was a happy one, with the nappy rash and cradle cap all cleared within two months.

Case 7: EM, male, age 36

This young man, employed as a local government officer, consulted me after seven years during which his health had declined dramatically. His major symptoms (and there were others) included bloating of the abdomen accompanied by nausea and flatulence, heartburn and indigestion. Constipation had become chronic. There was a tendency to lightheadedness and dizziness. He had periodic attacks of shivering followed by a high temperature which incapacitated him.

The onset of the condition, previous to which his health was unremarkable, came after an attack of gastroenteritis while on holiday. Treatment had, naturally enough, been with a broad-spectrum antibiotic. In his own words: 'For the 18 months following the gastroenteritis, I suffered all the symptoms daily, which were so severe, they resulted in my being unable to attend work for six months continuously, and the remaining 12 months, I attended only with massive support from my colleagues, who shared my workload, and understanding superiors, who allowed me to go home or rest when the attacks were extremely severe.'

There had been a gradual improvement over the following years until some 12 months prior to my seeing him when, after an acute attack, this young man was left with all the symptoms described above. At that time, he wrote, 'At present, I am struggling to cope with each day as it comes, and deal with this extremely debilitating and distressing illness as best I can.'

In the intervening years between the onset of his illness and consulting me, he had been seen by numerous medical practitioners. An endoscopy (at Charing Cross Hospital) showed no disease of the bowel. He was checked for what is called a 'malabsorption problem' but, again, no abnormality was found. He went to the Royal Homoeopathic Hospital on two occasions and consulted a herbalist, an osteopath and a medical specialist in allergies (a clinical ecologist). He had been placed on a rotation diet, which helped him to avoid repetitive contact with suspect food families, but had little effect on his condition.

At the time I first saw him, his diet was:

- Breakfast: *bacon* and tomato or *sausages*. Rice cakes and *marmalade*. Decaffeinated *coffee* and *fruit juice* (not freshly made)
- Mid-morning: fresh fruit
- Lunch: salad and baked potato plus *ham* or cottage cheese
- Evening meal: either *chicken* or *pork* or *sausages* or fish and vegetables.
- Bedtime: rice cakes and a hot *milk* drink before retiring.

(I have italicized those foods which are contraindicated in an anti-Candida diet.)

He appeared exhausted, but was a bright and intelligent patient who I felt would cooperate actively in any programme designed to assist his own recovery. After tests – including cytoxic tests to elicit specific foods to which he might be reacting and hair analysis (low in chromium, iron, manganese and selenium) – he was prescribed the following:

- An anti-yeast, anti-fungus pattern of eating, low in carbohydrates
- Supplements of vitamins A, E, B1, B2, B3, B6, calcium pantothenate (B5), calcium, magnesium and manganese. Vitamin C was also added. (The vitamin A was in emulsified form for easy absorption.)

- His pattern of eating was to include a seed and yoghurt breakfast, a salad lunch and an evening meal of 'safe' protein with vegetables.

At the time, our knowledge of biotin and acidophilus was not current and the above programme, which the reader will recognize as a modified version of that given in earlier chapters, had a remarkable effect. Improvement began soon after starting the programme. Two months later, biotin and acidophilus were introduced. Six months after the first visit, he reported at least a 50 per cent improvement in all symptoms; there were still some days of exhaustion but, overall, an upwards trend in his health was noted after seven years of decline. Confirmation of the involvement of Candida came with an attempt early in the programme to introduce an organic iron supplement in a liquid yeast-based form. This was met with an immediate return of constipation, which had more or less resolved itself. A check-up six months later found continued improvement, with lapses in the diet producing confirmatory flare-ups.

There is no reason to doubt that the condition will be kept under control and that the health of this patient will continue to improve. A letter just 18 months after the start of the programme states: 'Please accept apologies for delay in contacting you. It is an indication of the progress we have made that I am well enough not to have to adhere so strictly. I am very much better overall.'

Case 8: EV, female, age 50

This patient consulted me with a history of extreme itching and inflammation of the skin of the neck and scalp of one year's duration. She had an earlier history of acne, which was treated by antibiotic therapy (unsuccessfully).

She suffered from flatulence and had a history of colitis and a 'delicate' digestive system. She had consulted a herbalist, with little result, and a hypnotist, who taught her relaxation and helped her stop scratching the area, but the condition remained unchanged.

At the time of the consultation, I was not yet aware of the work of Dr Truss on Candida and my approach was to use nutrient supplementation based on her general clinical picture, a nutritional questionnaire, hair analysis and her current symptoms. Her dietary pattern was excellent (which, since this turned out to be a Candida problem, had probably saved her from far wider infestation).

She was placed on the following supplements, each taken orally: emulsified vitamin A, 60,000 IU; zinc orotate, 200 mg; calcium and magnesium orotates, 1 g each; chromium orotate, 10 mg; selenium, 50 mcg; oil of evening primrose (vitamin F), 1 g. I also suggested that she take yeast tablets as a source of vitamin B. At this point, she wrote to me (she lived a considerable distance from my practice) saying: 'I am following your suggestions carefully, except for the brewer's yeast. Over the years, I have tried a number of times to take it, but it creates gas and is most unpleasant.'

This set off alarm bells as I had just read the first of Dr Truss' articles that week. I immediately revised the pattern of eating which, while good under usual conditions, contained substances derived from yeast and, of course, a certain amount of 'yeast food' such as honey and muesli bars. The patient cancelled her following appointment with the comment that, as her symptoms had disappeared, she felt the journey unnecessary. A year later, she remained symptom-free, including both skin and bowel conditions.

Case 9: DB, female, age 31

DB, a computer programmer, had the following list of complaints:

- Eyes bloodshot and irritated for the past nine months
- Odd aches in joints and muscles
- Fingers slightly swollen
- Puffiness under the eyes (and sometimes above) after sleep.

Ten years since the onset of these symptoms, she had had cosmetic surgery and diuretics, but to no avail. She had been on a macrobiotic diet as well with no improvement. Her periods were erratic and painful, and her breasts became swollen and sensitive at this time. She felt unnaturally tired a good deal of the time. There was a history in her family of bronchial problems and depression, from which she also suffered.

Her current diet was:

- Breakfast: shop-bought *muesli with added sugar* plus *milk* or apple juice (once a week, she had eggs and *bacon* and *sausage* for breakfast)
- Lunch: a cooked vegetarian savoury or *sandwiches*
- Evening meal: fish and rice, occasionally meat.

During the day, she had the odd *candy bar* and three cups of *tea* plus *sugar* and *biscuits*. She had noticed a progressive inability to cope with alcohol. Her diet was reformed to remove the sugars and milk, and to increase complex carbohydrates. She was prescribed (after appropriate tests) vitamin B-complex, kelp, oil of evening primrose, vitamin B2, glutamic acid (an amino acid), and the minerals chromium, iron, manganese and selenium. Also prescribed were biotin and acidophilus, after meals. Within two months, she reported that her period had been on time for the first time in years, there had been a less overall tendency to swell (eyes or breasts) and she was able to cope with alcohol. (It was, in fact, proscribed from her diet, which raises the problem of patients' compliance with instructions, a major headache for practitioners.) Three months later, her condition was vastly improved, and her tiredness, blood-shot eyes, and aching muscles and joints had all diminished to a point where they no longer bothered her. A year later she was symptom-free.

Case 10: GH, female, age 29

The tragic progression of ill health in this case is a clear indictment of the failure of many health professionals to recognize Candida when it is staring them in the face. Before consulting me, GH wrote to me to say:

'I have been suffering from pelvic inflammatory disease (PID) for almost two years now. The problem started when I began to experience lower abdominal pain and feel generally unwell. I was, at the time, using the contraceptive IUD, which I had removed, believing this to be the cause of the pain. [Prior to this, it turned out, GH had been using the contraceptive pill, and had a history of recurrent thrush.] However, this [removal of the coil] had no effect and the pain became worse. Unfortunately, my GP did not diagnose PID, and I therefore received no treatment in the early stages of the disease. Eventually, I went to hospital, where the gynaecologist diagnosed PID through a laparoscopy. At that time, there was some damage to the fallopian tubes and adhesions in the pelvic area. I was put on antibiotics and, for a time, the condition seemed to improve. After a short time, however, I began to experience further attacks, and had to take larger doses of antibiotics regularly and strong painkillers for much of the time. At times, the pain was incredibly intense. In January 1983, I was admitted to a women's hospital in London for another laparoscopy. They found that both fallopian tubes were blocked, and it sounded as though damage/adhesions in the pelvic area had progressed. Despite this, I was told that the pain I was complaining of was psychological, and though they would be prepared to do tube reconstruction, for fertility purposes, there was nothing more they could do for me.

'I visited a consultant in Harley Street in February 1983, who said that my symptoms and pain were classic PID, but there was nothing he could do to help.

'My menstrual cycle had now gone from four to six weeks. Apart from the pain, other symptoms were active nausea, stomach upset, dizziness, a slightly raised temperature. I also became very depressed. In July 1983, I had surgery after consulting a leading gynaecologist at Hammersmith Hospital. This consisted of removal of the left fallopian tube and reconstruction of the right; separation of adhesions to tubes, ovaries and uterus through microsurgery; presacral neurotomy (removal of nerve to uterus); steroid treatment to prevent regrowth of adhesions.

'After this, all was well until early November 1983, when symptoms began again. Although pain was not as severe, tests showed the infection was active again. I was put on heavy doses of antibiotics. It did not clear up, and I am now in my sixth week of antibiotics. The consultant told me that there was nothing more they can do surgically and that I may have the condition for the rest of my life, and must learn to live with it. I have a very positive attitude towards getting better, and find it very difficult to believe that there is nothing else I can do to beat this disease, or at least fight it more effectively.'

This patient's history indicated that she had commenced on this sad slide to ill health at the age of 12, when cystitis was first apparent, after which she began a 13-year history of vaginal thrush. In late January 1984, this patient was placed on the programme as outlined in earlier chapters: high fibre, low refined carbohydrate, no fungal foods, and supplements of biotin, acidophilus, olive oil, zinc, vitamin F and garlic. Two months later, she reported that she was feeling considerably better, apart from a couple of bad spells from which she recovered more quickly than usual.

A letter dated 10 January 1985 reads:

'I have been feeling considerably better. The pain problem is now limited to a few days a month (around period time). After my last laparoscopy, the consultant said that it was the best result from that type of operation that he'd ever had. My remaining fallopian tube was tested and is clear, so I am a lot happier in myself.'

This is a clear and dramatic example of the tragedy that occurs when Candida becomes active in a young body, and of the effectiveness of the programme outlined in this book.

Conclusions

Candida is possibly the least understood, most widespread cause of ill health currently in our midst. Precisely because it is known to be everywhere, it is largely ignored and not even considered when a diagnosis of conditions, like that of GH (with PID), is sought. The cases quoted by Dr Truss, which include similar pictures to those described above, as well as individuals who were diagnosed as schizophrenic, manic-depressive and with multiple sclerosis deserve to be emphasized. All of these sufferers were restored to normality with the application of the sort of nutritional programme described in this book, together with anti-yeast drug treatment.

A wider awareness of this diagnosis as a possibility could very likely lead to a marked reduction in human suffering. Candida is not just a minor health irritant. It can destroy the physical and mental cohesion of an individual in a very short space of time. Prevention is by the same means as those described for treatment. The knowledge that we now have as to what makes Candida spread is easy to understand and easily put to practical use.

Self-help is always necessary and, until the medical profession becomes aware of the import of this knowledge, it is vital. Past experience in this regard is not comforting. It can take 50 years or more for an idea such as this one to permeate throughout the profession as a whole. Let us hope that, with modern forms of communication and the help of the media, this time lag will be speeded up in the case of Candida. The name of Dr C. Orian Truss, of Birmingham, Alabama, will eventually become well known throughout medicine. He is deserving of the gratitude of us all for his research into *Candida albicans* and its role as a cause of so much ill health.

REFERENCES

1 Werbach M, Murray M. *Botanical Influences on Illness*, Tarzana, CA: Third Line Press, 1996
2 Cappo B, Holmes D. 'Utility of prolonged respiratory exhalation for reducing physiological and psychological arousal in non-threatening and threatening situations', J *Psychosom Res* 1984; 28(4): 265–73
3 Ebringer A. 'The relationship between *Klebsiella* infection and ankylosing spondylitis', *Bailliere's Clinical Rheumatology*, 1989

Resources

Diagnostic test laboratories

Health Interlink
Asfordbury Business Park (Unit B)
Welby, Melton Mowbray
Leicestershire LE14 3JL
Tel: 01664 910 011
Practitioner needs to make initial contact

BioLab Medical Unit
The Stone House
9 Weymouth Street
London W1W 6DB
Tel: 020 7636 5959
Referral from physician required

Test kits for secretor status are available from

Stacktheme Limited
59 Bridge Street
Dollar
Clackmannanshire FK14 7DQ
Scotland
Tel: 01259 743 200
E-mail: info@stacktheme.com

Test kits to check for indoor mould contamination

Home Health Science
12 Wilson Drive
Sparta, New Jersey 07871
USA
Tel: +1 (877) 276 8250
E-mail: info@homehealthscience.com

Nutritional suppliers

The Nutri Centre
7 Park Crescent
London W1N 3HE
Tel: 020 7436 5122 or 020 7244 1138
The most comprehensive stock of nutrient and botanical products in the UK; will supply by post, and has resident nutritionists who can provide basic advice (relating to products) over the phone.

To locate practitioners specializing in Candida-related problems, use the directory in the following book

The Practical Guide to Candida
Author: Jane McWhirter
Publisher: All Hallows House Foundation
ISBN: 0952-6286-0-0
Tel: 020 7283 8908

Index

Also by Leon Chaitow

Fibromyalgia and Muscle Pain

YOUR SELF-TREATMENT GUIDE

Fibromyalgia is an increasingly common and now widely researched disorder. Sufferers experience widespread muscle pain and other associated symptoms such as chronic fatigue, disturbed sleep, bowel disorders, headaches, anxiety and PMS, yet it can be difficult to diagnose as many of the symptoms are similar to those of other illnesses.

This practical guide contains a range of self-tests and check-lists to help pinpoint symptoms, and looks at the value of various self-help measures to enhance recommended treatments, including:

- Massage and self-manipulation for muscle problems
- Hydotherapy, aromatherapy and acupuncture
- Detoxification and skin brushing
- Herbal and homoeopathic remedies and dietary advice
- Amino acids, antioxidants and other supplements
- Relaxation techniques for health enhancement

'Essential reading – not only for those who want to free themselves from these disorders, but also for loved ones and clinicians who want to help them to do so.'
Dr John C. Lowe, Director of Research, Fibromyalgia Research Foundation

BARBARA COUSINS

Cooking Without

Recipes free from added gluten, sugar, dairy products, yeast, salt and saturated fat, suitable for the control of weight, candida, chronic fatigue and allergies

Cooking Without is not only a collection of delicious and simple recipes but a book about health: how to gain it and how to keep it by giving the body the nutrients it needs to heal itself and stay well.

The recipes are flavoured with health-promoting ingredients rather than with high levels of salt, fat or sugar, and exclude wheat, dairy products and yeast, which are often linked to disorders such as candida and irritable bowel syndrome and can be an underlying factor in more serious health problems.

This book encourages you to build health by eating the right kinds of food at regular intervals, enabling the body to produce extra energy which can then be used for elimination, healing and weight control.

Barbara Cousins is a nutritional therapist who has been in practice for over 14 years. *Cooking Without* was written for her clients, and has achieved phenomenal success, helping thousands to enjoy better health and a better life.

BARBARA COUSINS

Vegetarian Cooking Without

Recipes free from added gluten, sugar, dairy products, yeast, salt and saturated fat, suitable for the control of weight, candida, chronic fatigue and allergies

Many vegetarian dishes rely on the use of milk, cream, cheese and wheat, and appetizing recipes without these ingredients are hard to find. In *Vegetarian Cooking Without* Barbara Cousins has put together a new collection of recipes which are not only for vegetarians, but for everyone wishing to include more healthy, enjoyable vegetarian meals in their diet.

Barbara's recipes are delicious, well-balanced and full of flavour, and include interesting new alternatives to gluten, dairy produce, sugar, yeast and saturated fat. The result is a way of eating that encourages the body to produce extra energy which can be used for healing, elimination and weight control.

Barbara Cousins is a nutritional therapist who has been in practice for over 14 years. Her first book, *Cooking Without*, was written for her clients, and has achieved phenomenal success, helping thousands to enjoy better health and a better life.

Make
www.thorsonselement.com
your online sanctuary

Get online information, inspiration and
guidance to help you on the path to physical
and spiritual well-being. Drawing on the integrity
and vision of our authors and titles, and with
health advice, articles, astrology, tarot, a
meditation zone, author interviews and events
listings, www.thorsonselement.com is a great
alternative to help create space and peace
in our lives.

So if you've always wondered about practising
yoga, following an allergy-free diet, using the
tarot or getting a life coach, we can point you
in the right direction.

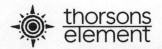

thorsons
element